Civil Rights Advocacy on Behalf of the Poor

American Governance: Politics, Policy, and Public Law

Series Editors: Richard Valelly, Pamela Brandwein, Marie Gottschalk, Christopher Howard

A complete list of books in the series is available from the publisher.

Civil Rights Advocacy on Behalf of the Poor

Catherine M. Paden

PENN

UNIVERSITY OF PENNSYLVANIA PRESS

PHILADELPHIA • OXFORD

Published by
University of Pennsylvania Press
Philadelphia, Pennsylvania 19104-4112
www.upenn.edu/pennpress

Printed in the United States of America on acid-free paper
10 9 8 7 6 5 4 3 2 1

Library of Congress Cataloging-in-Publication Data
Paden, Catherine M.
   Civil rights advocacy on behalf of the poor / Catherine M. Paden.
      p.   cm. — (American governance, politics, policy, and public law)
   Includes bibliographical references and index.
   ISBN 978-0-8122-4297-3 (hardcover : alk. paper)
   1. African Americans—Civil rights—Societies, etc.—History—20th century.   2. Social
advocacy—United States—History—20th century.   3. Civil rights movements—United
States—History—20th century.   4. Poor—United States—History—20th century.   5. Poor African
Americans—History—20th century.   I. Title.
E185.615.P26   2011
323.1196'073—dc22   2010018011

Contents

Chapter 1

Anti-Poverty as a Civil Rights Issue?

> I think certainly Katrina really underscored a real problem we've had in terms of
> black leadership . . . I'm talking about specifically black elected officials, black
> Democrats . . . and also the mainstream civil rights organizations: the NAACP,
> Southern Christian Leadership Conference, and, to an extent, the Urban
> League. . . . What we've seen . . . post-Katrina, during Katrina, and pre-Katrina
> . . . [is] a neglect of the African-American poor in terms of proactive policy
> initiatives, an active lobbying voice for a comprehensive program to deal with
> black poverty. What we're really talking about is a leadership that ignores, in
> terms of a comprehensive agenda, the poorest of the poor.
> —Earl Ofari Hutchinson, President, Los Angeles Urban Policy Roundtable,
> News and Notes with Ed Gordon, NPR, September 23, 2005

On August 28, 2005, Hurricane Katrina made landfall in New Orleans, eventually killing between fifteen hundred and two thousand people and leaving tens of thousands homeless. The images of New Orleans surprised some Americans, who were struck by the poverty there and that the majority of those affected were African American.[1] The disproportionate levels of poverty experienced by African Americans in New Orleans became front page news; media outlets displayed imagery of African Americans trapped in the city with no means for evacuation. In addition to exposing the ongoing intersection of race and poverty in the United States, Katrina made the distance between policymakers, elites, and the experience of low-income African Americans apparent. While touring the Houston Astrodome in the weeks following evacuation, former First Lady Barbara Bush remarked: "Everyone is so overwhelmed by the hospitality. And so many of the people in the arena here, you know, were underprivileged anyway, so this, this is working very well for them."[2]

As Americans scrambled to understand the impact of Katrina and to respond to the devastation, charitable organizations and advocacy groups swung into full gear raising money, finding volunteers, and offering commentary and explanations of the inequality Katrina brought to light. Among the active groups were civil rights organizations, which mobilized their membership, set up field offices in Louisiana and Mississippi, and made advocacy at the federal, state, and city levels a priority. This advocacy might not seem particularly surprising: given the conflation of race and poverty in the general perception, it may seem apparent that civil rights groups that are focused on racial equality would also advocate for the poor.[3]

However, as the quote at the beginning of this chapter reflects, representation of the poor has never been the top priority of civil rights organizations, which exist to eradicate racially prejudiced and discriminatory practices and policies. Literature on the activities and ideologies of civil rights groups argues that such organizations have functioned with a distinct middle-class bias since well before the 1960s civil rights movement (Goluboff 2007; A. Reed 1999; Marable 1985). Additionally, all political organizations face disincentives to represent the poor: such advocacy is expensive, politically unpopular, and often involves trade-offs with other issues that are more central to organizations' missions.

Nonetheless, because of the disproportionate effects of poverty on African Americans, civil rights groups have historically considered economic issues and issues of poverty to be inherently part of their missions. Although they varied in their chosen tactics and strategies, groups such as the Student Nonviolent Coordinating Committee (SNCC) and the Southern Christian Leadership Conference (SCLC) were particularly concerned with African American economic freedom.[4] Organizations and activists struggled to balance their commitment to sometimes radical economic goals with the necessity of working toward civil rights goals that were palatable to white liberals and policymakers (Jackson 2007). For many activists and leaders, the goals of civil rights were inseparable from those of economic equity because activists on the frontlines were struggling to overcome both racial and economic oppressions. As John Lewis, former SNCC chairman, explained:

> People have said that the civil rights movement was a middle-class movement. . . . But, a lot of the people that made up the rank and file of that movement, the people that got arrested and went to jail, the people

that participated in the marches, that stood in that immovable line, they were dirt poor.[5]

Additionally, middle-class African Americans might have particular interests in addressing issues of economic inequality. Research demonstrates that middle and upper class African Americans, who largely compose the membership of civil rights organizations, do not consider their own interests to be far removed from those of the African American poor. Scholars have found that African American middle-class status may be fragile—African Americans have less wealth and income than middle-class whites, and contend with housing segregation and discrimination as do the African American poor (Pattillo-McCoy 1999; Oliver and Shapiro 1995). Michael Dawson finds that shared interests based on race lead middle-class African Americans to care more about issues affecting the poor than their class status would predict (Dawson 1994).

Dawson's (1994) findings have spurred arguments about whether the emphasis on linked racial fate masks differences, and different interests, among African Americans. Although policy-makers and organizational leaders evoke linked racial fate with claims to represent "all African Americans," scholars have found that such claims are often accompanied by inactivity on behalf of nondominant subgroups. For example, Cathy J. Cohen (1999) finds that African American leadership largely neglected the disproportionate impact of HIV/AIDS on African Americans. Borrowing from her theory of primary and secondary marginalization, we could define organizational constituencies as either primary or secondary based on their level of marginalization within, and outside of, the organization (Cohen 1999). Often, the definition of a group's primary constituency is noncontroversial; it would be difficult to argue that the NAACP was not founded to represent African Americans. However, such broad identities are often difficult to translate into organizational priorities. Therefore, primary constituencies often dominate organizational priorities whereas secondary constituencies receive less attention, or are ignored altogether.

Additionally, advocacy that is considered to be relevant to an organization's overall constituency often carries implicit, and sometimes explicit, class biases. For example, civil rights organizations' relatively recent focus on affirmative action policies is interpreted by some scholars as the representation of middle-class interests, to the neglect of low-income African Americans (A. Reed 1999; Marable 1985). Skocpol argues that since the 1960s, professionally managed identity-based groups, such as civil rights organizations, have abandoned the interests of the poor and working classes, and solidarity across class lines has decreased (Skocpol 2003). In her Survey of National Economic and Social Justice Organizations, Strolovitch (2007) demonstrates that organizations claiming to represent "all African Americans" give disproportionate attention to issues affecting the wealthy and highly educated. She finds that civil rights organizations focus substantially more attention on affirmative action in higher education, an issue that affects an advantaged subgroup of their constituency, and less on welfare reform, an issue that affects a disadvantaged subgroup of their constituency (Strolovitch 2007, 121). These subpopulations often do not have the resources to establish their own organizations, and therefore are forced to rely on groups representing the broader constituency for possible representation of these specific interests (Robnett 2000). Therefore, whether civil rights organizations represent the poor is, in fact, an empirical question—such representation cannot be assumed.

This book examines civil rights organizations' levels of advocacy on behalf of the poor, shedding light on an important, yet largely unexamined, aspect of the groups' histories. Additionally, this research provides a unique opportunity to further understand the internal decision-making process of organizations—how do interest groups choose their priorities? What factors might lead groups to advocate on behalf of marginalized subpopulations of their constituencies? These questions allow for an assessment of the inclusiveness of American democracy, and shed light into an area of interest group scholarship that has not yet been adequately explored.

In following chapters, I examine five civil rights organizations and their decisions about whether to represent low-income African Americans during six legislative periods concerning welfare reform. Although scholars have studied the civil rights movement extensively, few have examined organizations' attention to anti-poverty policy, and none has assessed why groups chose to give priority to an issue that was secondary to their missions. One way to understand the decision-making processes of these organizations is to examine their archives, which provide the basis for an over-time comparison of organizational policy decisions and actions on behalf of the poor. I analyze the papers and archives of the Congress of Racial Equality (CORE), National Association for the Advancement of Colored People (NAACP), National Urban League (NUL), SCLC, and SNCC. I have also conducted interviews and corresponded with movement leaders and activists including former SNCC chairman John Lewis; Julian Bond, who was active with SNCC, SCLC, and NAACP; Bernard Lafayette, coordinator of the Poor People's Campaign (PPC) in 1968; and Hugh B. Price, former president and CEO of NUL. These interviews supplement my findings based on archival research, and provide a first-hand understanding of organizational decision-making from the decision-makers themselves.

The bulk of this book is an analysis of the activities of traditional civil rights groups concerning two pieces of welfare reform legislation intended to overhaul the welfare system: the 1964 Economic Opportunity Act (EOA) and the 1971 Family Assistance Plan (FAP). Because I seek to establish shifts in organizational priorities, I examine activities before the legislation was introduced, in support or opposition to the legislation while it was being debated, and after the legislation passed or died. Therefore, I assess organizational activities during four periods: the 1960–63 period captures state-led attempts to cut benefits and President John F. Kennedy's amendments to the Social Security Act; the 1964–65 period includes Lyndon Johnson's declaration of his "War on Poverty," the passage of the EOA in 1964, and the implementation of the Act in late 1964 and 1965; the 1966–68 period includes Congress's attempts to cut War on Poverty funding; and the 1969–72 period captures debate concerning the FAP.[6]

As the civil rights and welfare landscapes have certainly changed since the 1960s and 1970s, has advocacy by civil rights organizations evolved? I assess the activities of civil rights organizations in more recent anti-poverty battles based on public documents and interviews with leaders. Organizations varied in their responses to the needs of the poor during two very different battles—welfare reform during the mid-1990s and in response to Hurricane Katrina in 2005 and 2006. My findings indicate that civil rights organizations were largely inactive concerning the 1996 welfare reform bill. Although they participated in coalitions concerning President Bill Clinton's legislation, civil rights organizations did not take the lead in this advocacy. Alternatively, groups were active in response to Hurricane Katrina. In the months following the storm, local groups worked with national organizations to provide services for victims and advocate for increased federal assistance. However, once the national spotlight moved away from the storm, national advocacy decreased as well (see Table 1.1).

The case studies in this project concern periods when identity-based groups chose to represent the interests of particular subpopulations of their larger constituencies. In addition to its broader contribution to an understanding of organizational goal-setting, this project specifically examines how subpopulations are able to gain representation within identity-based groups. Traditionally excluded groups, including African Americans, gays and lesbians, and women, have developed effective advocacy organizations and have recently increased their political power through organizational representation and individual participation. However, within these identity-based groups, there are innumerable subpopulations, based on factors such as age, race, gender, national origin, and class, which are effected disproportionately by various policies

Table 1.1. Legislative Periods Examined

1960–1963	1964–1965	1966–1968	1969–1972	1994–1998	2005–2008
• State-led attempts to cut welfare spending • Kennedy amendments to Social Security Act	• Johnson declares War on Poverty • Economic Opportunity Act passed	• Amendments to EOA passed; first legislative cuts to War on Poverty spending	• Family Assistance Act introduced and debated	• TANF Reform (Personal Work Responsibility and Work Opportunity Reconciliation Act) and aftermath	• Response to Hurricane Katrina and aftermath

(Cohen 1999, 17; Strolovitch 2007). What factors determine whether these subpopulations gain organizational representation?

Who Gains Organizational Representation in the U.S. Political System?

Pluralists argue that competition among organizations allows multiple voices to be heard within the U.S. political system—power is dispersed among groups of citizens with common preferences and no one group of elites holds disproportionate levels of power (Truman 1960 [1951]; Dahl 2005 [1961]). Instead, groups and group leaders strive to attract members or ideological adherents. This creates competition among groups and ensures that all people have the opportunity to gain representation—some group leader will always be seeking their support. Because pluralist theory depends on competition within the political system, scholars pay attention to what types of groups exist, how groups form and maintain themselves, and who, in terms of group interest, is represented in the U.S. political system.

Each of these areas of scholarship is critical to understanding how organizations function within the U.S. political system; but such research rarely examines the internal dynamics and processes of groups.[7] Often, organizational goals and priorities have already been determined at the point when scholars examine organizational behavior. Although few scholars have analyzed the internal decision-making processes of organizations, many have noted the importance of such analysis.[8] Such an examination of how groups choose the issues, or interests, they will represent is central to a broader understanding of the U.S. political system.

In response to pluralists' celebration of the inclusiveness of American democracy, scholars have questioned whether the benefits of American government are available to all who seek them.[9] Given the impediments to individual participation, including time, money, and education, theorists argue that representation of politically marginalized groups is most likely to occur through interest groups (Berry 1984; Walker 1991). However, there are considerable disincentives to representing marginalized groups, such as the poor. Existing groups must be willing to advocate on behalf of a group that cannot contribute money to the organization and does not carry influence with policy-makers; groups concerned with the welfare of the poor must divert resources and attention away from service provision to political advocacy; or, new groups must be able to form and gain access to policy-makers (Walker 1991; Hays 2001). When representation of politically marginalized groups, such as the poor, does occur, it is therefore worthwhile to examine the factors contributing to the organizational prioritization of the groups' interest.

Civil Rights Advocacy on Behalf of the Poor moves beyond an understanding of such representation as very difficult, and sheds lights on how such advocacy may occur on issues affecting the poor. As I demonstrate, organizations that claim commitment to economic justice, among other issues, vary in their advocacy and approach to alleviating poverty. While an organization's claim to a commitment to economic justice may not be followed through with substantial advocacy at all, sometimes such a commitment becomes a group's top priority. The book provides an understanding of the various factors that lead some organizations to advocate on behalf of the poor, while not others.

Civil Rights Organizations' Advocacy on Behalf of the Poor

During the early and mid-1960s, civil rights groups were quite narrowly focused on passing the Civil Rights Act and Voting Rights Act, legislation intended to fight racial discrimination. After the passage of the acts, groups debated whether the movement should focus on overseeing their implementation or emphasize activities related to the goal of economic justice—a goal many groups and leaders saw as inseparable from civil rights, but which had taken a backseat to desegregation and nondiscrimination since the mid-1950s.[10] During this period, civil rights organizations, including the NAACP, relied heavily on membership contributions for revenue (Marger 1984).[11] As donations to civil rights groups dropped after 1965, the groups had little incentive to take on a politically unpopular priority that did not explicitly concern racial equality.[12] Declining membership numbers put organizations in precarious positions, and may have made a commitment to a costly goal, such as poverty alleviation, increasingly unattractive.[13]

Although literature on the activities and ideologies of civil rights groups has demonstrated a commitment to issues affecting the middle class, the literature also points to groups' dedication to advocacy concerning economic issues (Jackson 2007, 1993; Piven and Cloward 1977; Meier and Bracey 1993).[14] Charles Hamilton and Dona Hamilton (1997) argue that civil rights groups have consistently operated with a "dual agenda," focusing on both traditional civil rights issues as well as those concerning universal social policy.

> Civil rights organizations have consistently emphasized three main points: (1) preference for a universal social welfare system that does not distinguish between social insurance and public assistance, (2) jobs for all in the regular labor market, and (3) federal hegemony over social welfare programs (Hamilton and Hamilton 1997, 4).

Because they focus on universal and contributory social welfare policy, Hamilton and Hamilton (1997) do not examine organizational representation of public assistance recipients—an important distinction when discussing responses to social welfare policy. Public assistance policies are unique in the realm of social welfare because of their political unattractiveness; they are not publicly nor politically supported, and are not based on contributions from eventual recipients. Additionally, such policies have particularly affected women and children since their inception. As others have argued, welfare policy increasingly became a tool to control the sexual identity and behavior of African American women beginning in the late 1960s.[15] Civil rights organizations did not necessarily consider issues primarily affecting African American women to be their top priority.[16]

Additionally, African Americans were not the primary recipients of public assistance—in 1960, 40 percent of welfare recipients were African American.[17] Neither the Johnson administration nor the national media initially considered the War on Poverty particularly relevant to African Americans. Despite the inequitable nature of welfare disbursements, it was not until the War on Poverty that welfare policy came to be viewed through a racial lens and associated with African Americans (Lieberman 1998; Gilens 1999). In short, it was not at all obvious that the policy deserved a place on the race-centered agenda of civil rights organizations.

Even with these disincentives, my findings indicate that civil rights organizations chose to advocate on behalf of the poor throughout their histories. Some civil rights organizations increased their advocacy on behalf of low-income African Americans during the War on Poverty. The NAACP became involved at the national and local levels, and worked to increase its relevance to the African American poor. SNCC focused on grassroots organizing to ensure that low-income African Americans were not disempowered by the federal government's anti-poverty policy. CORE and the SCLC, on the other hand, did not substantially increase their advocacy on behalf of the poor until the late 1960s, when the War on Poverty programs came under attack. The organizations' differing conceptions of the importance of anti-poverty policy to their missions points to the inadequacy of relying on explanations such as federal funding being available for the implementation of the EOA, or the expectation that civil rights organizations would inherently have an interest in representing the poor.

My findings indicate that both structural factors, such as an organization's relationship with its local offices, and external factors, such as a group's relationship with other civil rights organizations, determined priorities. Each organization's response to external factors, such as competition with other civil rights organizations during the four legislative periods, was mediated by its internal structure and relations with local organizations. Groups sought to maintain their membership by staking out and guarding a unique position or niche among civil rights organizations. When leaders and staff perceived that advocacy on behalf of low-income African Americans would contribute to their organization's health and preeminence, such advocacy occurred. The form this advocacy took was mediated by an organization's structure, which determined groups' responses to anti-poverty policy.

Importantly, my findings indicate that a group's ideological commitment to economic justice does not necessarily lead to advocacy.[18] As I argue above, the costs of such representation, trade-offs with other issues that are considered to be more central to a group's overall mission and general constituency, and the political unpopularity of many economic justice issues provide strong disincentives to such advocacy. Even for SNCC, arguably the most ideologically driven group studied in this project, advocacy on behalf of the poor happened in part because of the group's acknowledgment of its effect on other civil rights organizations' priorities. Although a group's commitment to alleviating poverty certainly contributes to an organization's decision to pursue such goals, ideology does not tell us enough about when organizations pursue particular priorities. My findings that civil rights organizations varied in their attention to anti-poverty policy points to the fallacy of assuming that ideological commitment leads to strategic political action and advocacy.

Assessing Organizational Priorities

Determining organizational priorities, and the reasons groups arrive at those priorities, is a challenging task. Organizations have various audiences and means for expressing their priorities, and sometimes do not decide on an explicit hierarchy of goals. Archival research provides a unique opportunity to determine organizational priorities, and to assess the dynamics leading to internal decision-making within organizations. I examine materials such as annual reports, annual convention resolutions, speeches, and programs, internal memos, communications to membership, public speeches, and press releases. Both public and internal documents contribute to my assessment of organizational priorities and decision-making. For example, a program from an organization's national convention allows me to assess the amount of attention the group was devoting to anti-poverty policy; minutes from the board meeting where the convention was planned provides an understanding of the factors that contributed to determining the theme of the convention.

Interviews with former organizational leaders and staff contribute to my understanding of organizational approaches to anti-poverty policy.[19] I conducted open-ended, semistructured interviews with former leaders and current staff about their organization's consideration of the relevance of anti-poverty to civil rights (Aberbach and Rockman 2002, 674). When relevant, I asked about particular policies, such as the EOA of 1964, and organizational responses to that Act. The purpose of the interviews was to supplement my existing understanding of organizational decision-making; therefore, I did not ask leaders about details that would be difficult to remember with accuracy, such as the content of a particular meeting.

Because of its multiple case studies and reliance on archival research and interviews, this book sheds new light on *how* politically vulnerable groups are able to gain representation within the U.S. political system and moves beyond existing assessments of whether representation occurs. Other research points to the unequal representation of organizational constituencies—organizations privilege the representation of subgroups based on class, gender, and sexual orientation (Strolovitch 2007; A. Reed 1999; Cohen 1999). The research in this project illuminates when and how organizations depart from their usual focus on inequality to represent groups that they typically ignore, or whose concerns are often relegated to the margins of their advocacy work.

Additionally, much of the existing scholarship that assesses the goal-setting behavior of interest groups is unable to provide an in-depth understanding of decision making over time, and across organizations.[20] Surveys of interest groups offer snapshot understandings of organizational activities, but do not assess changes over time. Additionally, such surveys are limited to staff members' perceptions of organizational activities, and therefore often cannot assess overall priorities. Decisions to shift priorities rarely rest with an individual, and instead are organization-wide endeavors. A staff member may have an understanding of his or her role in implementing a group's goals, but may not be able to reflect on broader change within the organization. Reliance on archives allows the researcher to assess organizational activities across multiple departments. Additionally, comparative case studies across multiple organizations and time periods allow for an in-depth understanding of changes among, and within, organizations with similar missions and of the influence of dynamics among organizations on priorities and goals.

Explaining Organizational Priorities

Civil rights organizations are a particularly useful group to consider when assessing the influence of external and internal factors on decision-making because the organizations' internal structures, approaches to achieving social change, and commitment to political activity vary. For example, the NAACP and NUL were (and are) strongly bureaucratic organizations; SCLC was less bureaucratic, but very centralized; CORE was loosely federated; and SNCC struggled with its bureaucratic identity from its inception. Such differences among groups with similar missions facilitate analyses of how external and internal factors interact to affect decision-making within organizations and whether differences in structure determine the effect of external changes on priorities.

Increasingly, scholars recognize the importance of external factors and their effects on organizational decision-making.[21] The inclusion of external factors in models of organization decision-making takes different forms. The "new institutionalist" school of thought argues that the design of political institutions, and the rules that constrain them, are critical to understanding democratic systems. March and Olsen theorize that such institutions "define and defend values, norms, interests, identities, and beliefs" (March and Olsen 1989, 17). As applied to organizational behavior, scholars argue that instead of focusing on decision-making within an organization, it is important to examine institutional factors that define the universe of possible organizational goals and priorities (Berry and Arons 2003; Tarrow 1994; Walker 1991). Studies have also found that external factors define internal factors, such as rates of organizational growth, which in turn define priorities and goals (Gray and Lowery 1996). These two categories are not mutually exclusive; scholars argue that both types of effects of external factors are important to understanding organizational processes.[22]

Because of my reliance on archival materials, I am able to assess how organizations with varying structures respond to external factors when determining their priorities. Additionally, my analysis distinguishes the differing influences of external factors on priority-setting. For example, during the 1960s each civil rights organization may have considered itself to be in competition with other groups for membership. Did each organization feel this competition? How did competition affect priorities? Did the effect of competition vary based on organization structure? My findings indicate that each organization's response to such external factors during the four legislative periods was mediated by its internal structure and relations with local organizations.

Before assessing the factors that led to shifts in priorities, it is necessary to establish that such shifts occurred. In the next two chapters, I determine the level of attention each civil rights organization devoted to anti-poverty policy during the 1960s and early 1970s. Before presenting these findings, however, I introduce the organizations in the following section. An understanding of the similarities and differences among civil rights organizations is critical to any assessment of activities, and relationships, within the issue niche.

The Founding of Civil Rights Organizations, 1910–1960

The civil rights organizations analyzed in this project were founded to remedy prejudice and discrimination against African Americans. Despite their similar missions, each group was established with a distinct vision of how to achieve these broadly defined goals. Organizations faced varying political, social, and economic obstacles, contributing to each group's central purpose and means for achieving its goals. Additionally, each organization varied in governance structure, the role of membership, and overall bureaucratic nature. In addition to their founding principles, I highlight important structural features, which may influence organizational priorities.[23]

The Founding of Civil Rights Organizations in the Early Twentieth Century: NAACP and NUL

The NAACP was founded in 1910 to establish a permanent and lasting voice in the battle against lynchings, race riots, and unjust criminal prosecution of African Americans (Meier and Bracey 1993, 8). After several small meetings of white progressives, organizers invited African American organizers, lawyers, and social workers to join the small group, which continued to meet in New York City apartments until the National Negro Conference in 1909 (Kellogg 1967, 21). Participants in the first meeting of the National Negro Conference decided to found an organization with a permanent structure, including a public relations office, a legal committee, a political bureau, a civil rights commission, an education department, an industrial bureau, and an overseeing board (Rhym 2002, 34).

In 1910, the National Negro Committee changed its name to the National Association for the Advancement of Colored People and hired W. E. B. Du Bois as its first director of publicity and research. The Board passed the Constitution for Local Organizations Affiliated with the NAACP in 1911, establishing the goals the branches should pursue, as well as the role of the national office in relation to the branches.

> Activities of the branch were to include: the lessening of racial prejudice; the advancement of colored people; legal redress for colored persons unjustly persecuted; the setting up of a local bureau of information; mass meetings, parlor meetings, and memorial exercises; the study of local racial conditions; efforts to influence the press; efforts to lessen race discrimina-

tion and to secure full civil rights and political rights to colored citizens and others; and the establishment of a civic center for the work. The local program was in the hands of the branch, but general policy was under control of the parent organization. (Kellogg 1967, 120)

The NAACP was founded as a highly bureaucratic organization that would be governed by membership through representation at the organization's annual conventions. The annual convention was open to participation by any youth council, college chapter, and local branch that had maintained the minimum membership requirements to be granted a charter by the national office. Policies and positions were determined by the annual convention, which then governed the Board of Directors, branches, youth councils, and any other subunits of the NAACP.[24] Although local offices were allowed to determine their own strategies for attracting membership and influencing policy through legislatures and the courts, all decisions and priorities on the part of branches had to be first approved by the national office. If the Board of Directors disagreed with the activities of local branches, branches were required to abide by the Board's decision.

The national office has worked to maintain its control over potential, and existing, branch offices since the organization's founding. According to the 1911 bylaws, applications for affiliation were to be submitted to, and approved by, the National Board of Directors. Each branch was under the authority of the National Board, and the organization's bylaws stipulated that the Board must approve of each branch's constitution (Kellogg 1967, 119). The national office received the majority of all dues collected by the branches, although the local offices kept a small portion to pay for their own expenses. Branches were allowed to raise money through other means, and to keep all proceeds from this fundraising. Each local unit was required to report on its activities through a monthly report to the national office, and the executive secretary of the national office was responsible for communicating to each branch via a monthly newsletter (Kellogg 1967, 91).

The bylaws were revised in 1914, 1915, 1916, 1917, and 1918, expanding the number of Board members to forty and revising residency requirements for Board members, among other changes. During this period, financial stability was an overriding concern of the board. As the NAACP expanded, its expenses grew without means for proportionately increasing the organization's income. The organization relied on contributions from Board members for its income, which were often sporadic and difficult to count on. In 1914, more than half of the organization's income came from eighteen contributors (Kellogg 1967, 106). The organization's financial difficulties forced it to concentrate its efforts on attracting contributors outside of the Board, as well as to begin to consider membership outreach programs.

Beginning in 1916, the Board began to discuss the expansion of NAACP membership, both numerically and geographically, and emphasized the importance of maintaining national office control over the branches. In 1918, the organization embarked on an intense membership drive through the national office, as well as its branch offices (Kellogg 1967, 120). The newly created Department of Branches, and its director, Mary White Ovington, contributed to the effectiveness of this drive, as did the heightened racial consciousness of Americans generally during World War I. During this period, an extensive migration of blacks to northern cities began, race riots were common, the Ku Klux Klan was revived, Marcus Garvey and his United Negro Improvement Association began to attract membership and attention, and the Harlem Renaissance began—all of which contributed to a heightened racial consciousness among African Americans. By 1920 membership dues from African Americans supplied most of the organization's income. At the same time that black membership was increasing, the NAACP was performing outreach to sympathetic whites (Kellogg 1967, 134).

The NAACP's goals during the period after its founding focused on securing liberty for African Americans through anti-lynching legislation, criminal defense in cases resulting from the race riots in U.S. cities during the early twentieth century, and equitable criminal representation in general. As opposed to the political focus of the NAACP, the NUL was founded as an organization relying on social work and the distribution of social services. In fact, the organization did not engage in political activities until the 1940s (Moore 1981, 48). To open up industrial job opportunities for African Americans, three organizations were merged to establish the National League on Urban Conditions Among Negroes (NLUCAN) in 1911, which would later become the NUL: the Committee on Urban Conditions Among Negroes in New York, the Committee for Improving the Industrial Conditions of Negroes in New York, and the National League for the Protection of Colored Women (Parris and Brooks, 1971).

Unlike the founders of the NAACP, the African Americans involved in the formation of NLUCAN did not insist on a goal of social equality between African Americans and whites. Many whites involved in the founding believed that social equality was a private matter, and should not be decided through the courts or legislation. The ideologies of the founders varied, but they agreed that African Americans living in U.S. cities should have equal access to economic and political opportunities.

Uniting the Negro and white NUL founders was the belief that the problems spawned by industrial and social unrest and by class conflicts and class enmities affected society as a whole. Unless these problems were resolved, the NUL founders concluded . . . America . . . faced a dire and uncertain future." (Moore 1981, 47)

From its founding, the NUL established its role as a social work and social service agency. The organization's first executive director, George E. Haynes, and its first Board of Directors, agreed that NUL's role in the advancement of racial equality should be "To carry on constructive and preventive social work among Negroes . . . to bring about coordination and cooperation between existing agencies . . . to secure and train Negro social workers."[25] The organization also focused upon studying urban conditions scientifically, and believed that such studies would provide solutions to social, economic, and political disparities faced by African Americans in northern cities (Moore 1981, 55).

In 1911, the same year as the national organization's founding, Eugene K. Jones, a social worker, was named as the organization's first field secretary. Due to financial necessity, the national organization was interested in establishing local affiliates in additional northern and southern cities. However, to become an affiliate, a group first had to qualify as a member of a Community Chest, taking the financial burden off of the national office as it established affiliates.[26] The National Board did not rush to establish affiliates, but rather preferred to wait until the local group could demonstrate its financial independence from the national organization (Moore 1981, 57). Nonetheless, the national office authorized twenty-seven affiliates by 1918. By 1961, the League had grown to sixty-six affiliates (Dickerson 1998, 38). Unlike NAACP affiliates, NUL affiliates were highly autonomous and were responsible for determining their own programming. Additionally, the NUL did not function as an individual-based membership organization. The League's affiliates were considered its members.

The Founding of Civil Rights Organizations in the Mid-Twentieth Century: CORE, SCLC, and SNCC

While the NUL focused on industry negotiations and social service during the 1940s, a group of pacifists established an activist organization to fight racial discrimination, CORE, which was founded in Chicago in 1942. CORE was created as an interracial organization committed to nonviolent strategies (Meier and Rudwick 1975 [1973], 6). CORE primarily functioned as an intellectually oriented organization; its few members were focused on combating racial discrimination based on philosophical understandings of justice and freedom, not through mass actions (Morris 1984, 129). The circumstances of CORE's founding had lasting implications for the organization.

During the early to mid-1950s, CORE's activities to fight discrimination were largely unknown by African Americans, and even among civil rights activists. The organization was not mass-based; its small number of local offices consisted of five or six members who would periodically protest racial discrimination. James Farmer, who would become CORE's director in 1961, emphasized that the organization largely appealed to white middle-class intellectuals who were committed to nonviolence, and were seeking the means to achieve social justice without violent confrontations. Before the late 1950s, CORE believed that using nonviolent resistance in the South would be fruitless—the discriminatory barriers would be too difficult to penetrate. However, after leadership began to see nonviolent protests by blacks in the South, it decided that CORE should become active in the area. The organization viewed itself as particularly suited for nonviolent organizing, since it was the basis of its founding (Morris 1984, 130).

CORE's interest in expanding into the South was facilitated through its hiring of James McCain as its first field secretary. McCain, an African American Morris College graduate who had been president of the local NAACP chapter, was particularly suited to increase CORE's visibility among African Americans in the South. By 1958, he had established seven CORE groups in South Carolina, which would be vital to the organization's attention to, organization of, and participation in the sit-ins that began in 1960 throughout North and South Carolina (Morris 1984, 133). Throughout 1960, CORE increased its visibility within the South, and among other civil rights organizations, through the sit-in movement. CORE named nonviolent, direct action as its only method to achieve social change, and indicated that its members would readily cooperate with other groups, provided that those groups adhered to CORE's commitment to interracial nonviolent direct action.[27]

The national office considered its role to be one of a coordinating agency for local CORE groups. The national office's function was to support and publicize the activities of local affiliates, and to represent such activities at the national level through congressional lobbying. However, the national office did not embark on activities separate from those of its affiliates.[28] The election of James Farmer, who had become a visible and charismatic leader during the sit-ins, as the organization's national director on February 1, 1961, indicated the organization's commitment to further increasing its visibility within the burgeoning civil rights movement, and its commitment to mass-action among African Americans.

During 1961, CORE organized the Freedom Ride, which catapulted the organization into the national spotlight, and secured its position of preeminence among civil rights organizations. The Ride left Washington, D.C., on May 4, 1961 to: "penetrate the deep South . . . focus on [transportation] facilities . . . the riders . . . pledge[d], if arrested, to remain in jail rather than accept bail or pay fines" (Meier and Rudwick 1975 [1973], 136). Once the riders entered Alabama, they faced mob violence and mass arrests. Because of the violent responses to the Ride, CORE received national attention as a mass-based civil rights organization. This attention led to a jump in CORE's income, allowing the organization to rapidly expand throughout the North and South. Additionally, it marked the first time that CORE had mobilized working-class African Americans, marking a shift away from the organization's reputation as elitist (Meier and Rudwick, 145).

The SCLC was founded in Atlanta, Georgia, on January 11, 1957. Similar to CORE, the SCLC's founding principles included nonviolence and interracialism. Rev. Dr. Martin Luther King, Jr., Rev. Fred L. Shuttlesworth, Rev. C. K. Steele, and Rev. T. J. Jemison convened a group of Southern religious leaders to respond to the rising levels of protests among African Americans in the South. Although African American women, including Ella Baker who was one of the founders of the organization, were high-ranking staff members of the SCLC, there was no question but that the ministers would be the organization's leaders and spokespeople. As Baker explained:

> There would never be any role for me in a leadership capacity in the SCLC. Why? First, I'm a woman. Also, I'm not a minister. . . . The combination of the basic attitude of men, and especially ministers, as to what the role of women in their church set ups is—that of taking orders, not providing leadership. . . . This would never have lent itself to my being a leader in the movement there.[29]

Initially, the organization was founded as a coordinating agency among local organizations engaged in registration and integration activities (Garrow 1986). The SCLC's founding established it as a coordinator of local community organizations:

> The SCLC is organized as a service agency to facilitate coordinated action of local protest groups and to assist in their sharing of resources and experiences. . . . The SCLC seeks to cooperate with all existing agencies attempting to bring full democracy to our great nation.[30]

Generally, the language of the organization's bylaws does not advocate for particular programs or policies—most concern the role of Christian ministers in the organization and the goal of interracial cooperation. However, the means of working with national, state, and local agencies is emphasized in both the Constitution and bylaws. Coordination with existing agencies was a priority in the "Aims and Purposes" section of its Constitution and was discussed in every one of the seven articles of the bylaws. Specific means for working with existing agencies are not discussed; however, it is clear that the SCLC was founded to coordinate existing efforts in the South to disable Jim Crow segregation.[31]

Despite its mission at its inception, of being a facilitating agency among local organizations, the SCLC would eventually establish a highly coordinated network of affiliates, directed by the national office. Such changes in organizational structure have had implications for the policy issues prioritized by the group. For example, the Department of Affiliates at the national office was established to coordinate efforts among local organizations, and to be sure that the overall movement was prioritizing the same concerns, specifically voter registration. Eventually, this local/national coordination would be the basis for the national office's organization of the PPC in 1967 and 1968.

Soon after its founding, the SCLC launched its Citizen Education Project, running workshops throughout the South to inform African Americans of their voting and political participation rights and responsibilities. The founders considered access to political power to be critical to gaining civil rights throughout the South; therefore, barriers to full participation required organizational response. The SCLC commitment to social change through political participation drove the organization's attention to the issue of economic inequality, and its priority of mobilizing the poor in the late 1960s.

The SNCC was founded in 1960 to coordinate the activities of student protestors throughout the South. Ella Baker, executive director the SCLC, convened SNCC's founding meeting in April 1960 to organize the students who had been coordinating sit-in protests (Carson 1995, 19). Consistent with the SCLC's ideology, SNCC's original statement of purpose included the organization's commitment to nonviolence as a political tactic: "We affirm the philosophical or religious ideal of nonviolence as the foundation of our purpose. . . . Through nonviolence, courage displaces fear; love transforms hate. Acceptance dissipates prejudice; hope ends despair. . . . Justice for all overthrows injustice."[32]

SNCC was not founded as a permanent organization—the founding meeting established a temporary coordinating committee for student activists. It was not until its fall conference in October 1960 that SNCC gained permanent organizational status. The October conference created the permanent coordinating committee and emphasized the importance of local groups retaining their autonomy. "Coordination in each state . . . is recognized as necessary for greater effectiveness, but there is no concentration of centralization of authority. Authority rests with local groups of students."[33] In addition to maintaining the autonomy of local groups, the conference stated SNCC's independence from other civil rights organizations: "The SNCC shall remain self-directing but shall welcome cooperation with adult organizations which are support-ing the movement."[34] Because of this founding principle of establishing independence from the traditional civil rights organizations, African American women were initially more likely to serve in leadership posi-tions in SNCC (Giddings 1984, 277). Autonomy and self-direction were guiding principles for the organization, and became organizing princi-ples for SNCC activists working in low-income rural communities: Afri-can Americans should strive for self-sufficiency, and not rely on national organizations, or the federal government, for social, political, or eco-nomic improvements.

As these brief histories illustrate, and as Table 1.2 summarizes, each civil rights organization was founded with its own purposes and ideol-ogy. During the 1960s these organizations worked together to achieve common goals, but remained distinct groups with differing tactics and goals. These differences are critical to understanding why each group chose to advocate on behalf of the poor. In the next two chapters, I establish when each organization chose to prioritize anti-poverty policy. The remainder of the book assesses the factors that led organizations to shift the level of attention they devoted to advocacy on behalf of the poor.

Plan of the Book

In the next chapter, I introduce my data and methods for assessing and analyzing shifts in organizational priorities. Based on an examination of existing theoretical explanations for decision-making, as well as litera-ture specific to the representation of marginalized groups, I present my model of organizational decision-making. In Chapters 3 and 4, I present case studies of civil rights organizations during periods when they shifted their level of advocacy on behalf of the poor. In Chapter 5, I analyze organizational responses to the War on Poverty during the mid- to late 1960s. Based on this analysis, I argue that older, more established civil rights organizations shifted their priorities based on the anti-poverty activities of newer, more radical organizations. Each organiza-tion's level of advocacy on behalf of the poor varied based on the national groups' structures, and their relationships within the civil rights issue niche.

In Chapter 6, I present the case studies of organizational responses to the proposal of the FAP in 1969. Although less than a decade after the War on Poverty legislation, the early 1970s was a period of upheaval for

Table 1.2. Founding of Civil Rights Organizations

Organization	Year founded	Founding purpose/goals	Relevant structural attributes
National Association for the Advancement of Colored People	1910	• Anti-lynching legislation • Criminal justice	• Highly bureaucratic organization • Annual convention resolutions determine organizational priorities • National control over local offices
National Urban League	1911	• Social service provision • Coordination of local social service providers	• Highly bureaucratic organization • Autonomous local offices determine their own activities in line with national office priorities
Congress of Racial Equality	1942	• Nonviolent protest • Intellectual roots in pacifism	• Loosely structured organization • Small number of local offices; few active members
Southern Christian Leadership Conference	1957	• Coordination of Christian ministers • Nonviolent protest • Mass action	• Structured organization • Nationally directed local offices
Student Nonviolent Coordinating Committee	1960	• Coordinating committee for student protest groups • Nonviolent protest • Mass action	• Intentionally nonstructured organization • Intentionally weak direction of student groups by national office

both older and newer civil rights organizations. All groups faced declines in membership and income. Established organizations were uninterested in the more radical groups' embrace of black power ideologies. As opposed to the mid-1960s, these radical groups saw membership and funding decline. As the more radical organizations became less of a threat to the older groups, the latter did not feel pressure to expand their constituencies to include the poor. Although new organizations, such as the National Welfare Rights Organization (NWRO), were founded to represent the interests the poor, civil rights organizations did not consider these groups to be competition for membership because they were outside the civil rights niche. Civil rights groups were active concerning the FAP, but the plan was less of a priority than the War on Poverty programs had been less than a decade before.

In Chapter 7, I discuss civil rights organizations' involvement in more recent anti-poverty battles. Based on analysis of organizational participation in congressional hearings and interviews with leaders and legislative staff, this chapter assesses organizational activities concerning the 1996 welfare reform bill and the response to Hurricane Katrina in 2005 and 2006. Additionally, interviews with leaders and staff explore organizations' overall attention to issues affecting low-income African Americans, and how leaders and staff conceive of their missions as they relate to issues of poverty. During the 1990s, groups focused on their own well-being and survival without incentives to become engaged in welfare reform. In response to Hurricane Katrina, on the other hand, groups rose to a national call for advocacy on behalf of the poor. Once that call subsided, civil rights advocacy declined.

My research demonstrates that the interaction between internal and external factors will determine organizational priorities. An organization's response to external factors, such as the activities of other groups in its issue niche, is mediated by internal factors, such as its structure. Therefore, my findings indicate that organizational decision-making cannot be understood without an examination of both internal and external factors. In Chapter 8, I draw conclusions about what factors contribute to an organization's decision to substantially shift its priorities, and how the poor gain representation in the United States. I explore the possibilities for, and the barriers to, increasing democratic inclusion in U.S. politics and policy-making through interest group representation.

Chapter 2

Assessing and Explaining Shifts
in Organizational Priorities

MEMBERSHIPS ARE N[umber] 1. No matter what successes the NAACP Branches have had in meeting local problems, the general public over the nation will judge the whole NAACP . . . by one question: "Did the total membership go up or down?" . . . If it goes up, the NAACP is a going concern. . . . If it goes down, the NAACP is dying on its feet. You know that is not a fair way to judge, but that is how it is today. The newspapers, the editorial writers, the columnists, the radio and TV commentators will judge the NAACP by the total membership. You know you did a good job in your city and state on several projects. You know you have backed the national program. . . . But they go by memberships. So—you must go by memberships.

    —Roy Wilkins, NAACP Executive Director, to NAACP branch and Youth
    Council leaders, September 28, 1966

Before exploring why civil rights organizations advocated on behalf of the poor during some periods and not others, it is necessary to establish when, and to what extent, such advocacy occurred. When did civil rights organizations shift their level of attention to representation of the poor? As I discuss in the previous chapter, my analysis of organizational decision-making is based on the archives of five civil rights organizations: CORE, NAACP, NUL, SCLC, and SNCC.[1] After explaining my approach to assessing priority shifts, I discuss why these shifts may have occurred. I then present my theoretical expectations about the factors that may lead organizations to shift their priorities. Finally, I present my model of decision-making based on existing literature on interest group decision-making.

Method: Establishing and Explaining Shifts

Establishing Shifts in Organizational Priorities

Sometimes it is clear when an organization is prioritizing an issue—local affiliates are mobilized, organizational representatives make public speeches, and media attention is focused on the organization's activities. Such an impressive campaign on an issue gains publicity for the organization spearheading the effort, and can be quite beneficial for the group in the long-term. In the short-term, however, it is quite costly. Only an organization that is financially comfortable and has a presence in multiple states or urban areas, access to media attention, and the ability to attract participants to public gatherings could conceive of such a campaign. Smaller organizations, or even large ones that do not wish to devote all of their resources to one issue, may prioritize advocacy on issues without embarking on an all-consuming campaign.

To determine shifts in organizational priorities, it is necessary to measure the level of priority each organization devoted to anti-poverty policy during distinct time periods. However, quantifying an organization's level of commitment to an issue is not simple. Organizations engage in many different types of activities, and for many different reasons. Factors distinct to each organization, such as whether it generally relies on direct action tactics, mobilizes local organizations, or has local branches, will affect how it prioritizes an issue. As Table 2.1 illustrates, I have included various types of activities at each level of priority.[2]

According to my scales of priority, indicators of an organization's high level of commitment to an issue include explicit statements of the issue as an organizational priority, internal structural changes aimed to make the organization's activities concerning the issue more effective, and activities that involve the mobilization of membership, or an organization's constituency. These reflect an organizational commitment to the issue that is financial, but also involves membership. Without some evidence of membership involvement, an organization's commitment to an issue is not classified as a high priority.

When the NUL decided to make the War on Poverty a high priority, it underwent organizational restructuring: it notified its affiliates of the new organization-wide priority, retrained affiliate leaders to work with and advocate on behalf of low-income African Americans, and worked

Table 2.1. Organizational Activities as Indicators of Priority

Low-priority indicators (1 point each)
• Position taken on issue (statement, convention resolution)

Mid-level priority indicators (2 points each)
• Staff, or organizational committee, assigned to issue as one of several, or only, assignments
• Internal evidence of funding for activities concerning issue
• Communications to policy-makers about issue (testimonies before Congress or parties, position letters)
• Public speeches or statements by staff/leadership about issue
• National office directs local branches/affiliates to be active on issue
• Mailings to membership about issue

High-level priority indicators (3 points each)
• Fundraising with membership about issue
• Mobilization of membership for actions about issue
• Consultation with policy-makers about issue (legislative drafting, implementation)
• National office offers workshops/training for local branches/affiliates on issue
• Internal discussions, as reflected in meeting minutes and transcripts, indicate issue as priority
• Organizational documents name issue as priority (resolutions, annual reports, organizational publications)
• Organizational restructuring to address issue (overall restructuring, creation of new department)
• Organization offers own plan concerning issue

No evidence of priority
• Absence of any evidence of issue as priority

in close contact with the White House and members of Congress in the implementation of the poverty program. An example of evidence of anti-poverty policy being a high priority for the organization is found in its report on the resolutions and recommendations passed by the 1964 annual conference. The document describes the workshops held for NUL branch leaders, and other relevant civil rights leaders, about implementation of the War on Poverty.[3] When I assessed the NUL commitment to the War on Poverty, these workshops counted as high priority indicators, and were included as evidence of "National Office offers workshops/training for local branches/affiliates on issue."

At a mid-level commitment, a group has allocated ongoing resources and staff to the issue, but has not reached out to membership through direct mobilization. A group devoting a mid-level of commitment does not extend its activities outside of the national or Washington office. Staff may testify before congressional committees or political parties

about the issue, but will not activate membership to contribute funds
for activities on the issue, or to participate in demonstrations. During
the mid-1960s, the NAACP devoted a mid-level of attention to the War
on Poverty. At a Board of Directors meeting in September 1964, the
Board discussed how to get involved. Minutes from the meeting reported that the executive director emphasized the importance of the
War on Poverty as a direction for the NAACP, and that the national
office should figure out how to work at the local level to implement the
anti-poverty legislation.[4] I coded this information as evidence of "Internal discussions, as reflected in meeting minutes and transcripts, indicate
issue as priority," an indicator of a high level of attention being devoted
to anti-poverty policy. However, because the NAACP did not mobilize its
membership or branches on the War on Poverty, its cumulative activities
reveal a mid-level of attention to poverty issues.

If an issue is a low priority for an organization, the group may offer
rhetoric either supporting or opposing a policy, but will not commit any
substantial organizational resources, in terms of staff or funding, to it.
For example, a staff member may attend a coalition meeting about a
piece of legislation, but that will be the staff member's only activity concerning the legislation. Coalition activity itself might indicate various
levels of organizational commitment to an issue. As Strolovitch (2007)
finds, coalition activity is particularly relevant for organizations engaged
in policy battles, like welfare reform, that cut across multiple identities,
such as race, class, and gender. If an organization actively participates in
a coalition, activities such as fundraising and membership mobilization
indicate a high commitment to the issue, based on my priority scales. On
the other hand, staff attendance at a coalition meeting requires minimal
organizational resources. The most common low-priority activity among
the groups was to pass convention resolutions or statements concerning
the War on Poverty. In fact, all of the civil rights organizations did so. I
counted such statements as low-priority indicators, "Position taken on
issue (statement, convention resolution)."

My methodology allows me to present archival information in a stan-
dardized form, providing an understanding of fluctuations in attention
to anti-poverty policy, both across and within organizations. For each
low-level priority indicator, I assign a group one point; for each mid-
level priority indicator, a group receives two points; and, for each high-
level priority indicator, a group receives three points. I then determine
the organization's activities as a percentage of total possible activities.
Once fluctuations in priorities are documented, it is possible to examine
why shifts in organizational attention to the poor occurred, contributing
to an understanding of organizational decision-making, and to an
awareness of how politically marginalized groups gain representation.

To facilitate comparisons among organizations, each type of activity only counts once in my determination of priority level. This approach allows me to take into account differences in organizational resources. The NAACP may send one mailing, or five mailings, to its branches concerning anti-poverty policy. I am not counting how often the activities occur, but rather what types of activities occur. A variety of activities concerning an issue indicates organizational commitment to it. Judging commitment to an issue based on the number of times a group engages in a particular activity would benefit larger organizations. Simply because an organization sends five mailings to branches does not indicate that the organization is, overall, committed to the issue. The branch department may be the only component of the organization working on it. A group that produces four organizational brochures naming an issue as a priority may be no more committed to it than a group that produces one brochure but sends it to its entire membership and policy-makers. Assessing the variety of activities an organization devotes to an issue provides a nuanced understanding of the type and level of attention it received.[5]

Evaluating the Factors That Influence Organizational Decision-Making

Once I am able to determine that organizations shifted their priorities, I seek to explain these shifts. To determine the factors that led to priority change, I categorize potential factors as either internal or external to the organization. This division is somewhat artificial; the relationship between an organization and its external environment cannot be neatly separated (Gray and Lowery 1996). For my purposes, this division is used to simplify coding, but does not affect my analysis of the relationship between internal and external variables. For each variable examined, I analyze materials in each organization's archives including annual reports; annual convention resolutions, speeches, and programs; internal memos, communications to membership, public speeches, press releases, and organizational documents. I assess the impact of each document based on its content, author, and intended audience. For example, a memo from a national field director to an executive director about the problems with expanding branch activity indicates that these problems existed, and that the national office was responding to them. On the other hand, a similar letter from a branch officer to the national office does not indicate that the national office found such concerns to be pressing, or was responding to them.

I evaluate the relationship between the independent variables and an organization's attention to welfare reform in two ways. First, I determine the role of the independent variables during a time that the organization is focusing on welfare reform. For example, the SCLC prioritized anti-poverty issues during its mass campaign fighting welfare reform policies. This was a shift in priority after the victories of the Civil Rights and Voting Rights Acts, and occurred after several months of internal discussions. Based on internal and external documents, membership numbers, budget numbers, branch numbers, and reorganization activities, I determine changes in the independent variables during the period before the planning of the anti-poverty campaign. While this method does not establish a causal relationship between changes in an organization's structure and its attention to welfare policies, I am able to draw conclusions because I examine the influence of structural changes on multiple organizations, over multiple time periods.

Second, in many cases, the content of resolutions, speeches, and internal memoranda divulge reasons for the organization's attention to the issue. For example, a memo from an executive director to his or her assistant stating that the organization must begin to focus on public assistance issues to attract the support of the masses indicates the importance of a group's constituency to its determination of priorities. In the quote below, Roy Wilkins, executive director of the NAACP, explains to branch leaders that the NAACP should increase its attention to the War on Poverty to maintain its preeminence within the civil rights movement:

> As one of the Association's leaders, you will recognize at once that we are striking out in a new direction and launching a major new program area [the War on Poverty]. You will also, I believe, welcome it as an absolutely necessary move if the Association is to maintain its leadership in our movement.[6]

Such documents, which present apparently causal reasoning, establish the relationships between the independent variables and the organization's attention to poverty, and help tell the story of the organizational changes and their effects on the organization's emphasis on welfare issues. However, simply because a reason for a priority shift is given in an organizational document does not indicate that other factors were not also relevant. I assess organizational explanations for shifts in focus, but also take into account the presence of other internal and external factors that may have contributed to them. In the next sections, I present my expectations of how internal and external factors interact to determine organizational priorities.

What Factors Determine Organizational Priorities?

After establishing in the next two chapters that organizations shifted their levels of attention to anti-poverty policy, I present in Chapters 5 and 6 my findings as to why these shifts occurred. Overall, I argue that organizations determine their priorities based on their perceptions of what goals will contribute to their maintenance, and possibly their growth (Wilson 1995 [1973]). Organizations whose main purpose is to achieve defined ideological goals, or purposive organizations, determine their health based on their relationship with their membership, or constituency. A purposive organization's membership will contribute financially to the organization, therefore contributing to its overall health. More importantly, however, policymakers, foundations, and government agencies determine an organization's viability based on its membership numbers.

We know a great deal about the influence of membership on groups from existing literature. When an organizational leader, or a group's board, is determining priorities, the preferences of existing membership will certainly be considered (Moe 1980; Rothenberg 1992), as will the preferences of the group's potential membership or constituency (Truman 1960 [1951]). What is less established, however, are the factors that determine how a leader, or board, assesses the preferences of an organization's existing, or future, constituency when determining priorities. It is unlikely that an organization's membership shares a common set of interests. Particularly among identity-based groups, divisions within the group based on class, gender, sexual orientation, or a host of other factors may create distinct interests among subgroups within an organization's overall membership (Cohen 1999; Strolovitch 2007). Given the varieties of interests within an organization's constituency, how does a group determine whose interests it will represent? My findings indicate that both internal and external factors influence an organization's perception of which activities will contribute to its well-being, and therefore, which issues will become its priorities.

Purposive Organizations' Concern with Membership

The decisions about the goals an organization will pursue rest with its leadership, staff, governing board, and, rarely, its membership. Although organizations may signal to members that their opinions about organizational priorities matter through surveys and membership meetings, scholars have found that opinions of rank-and-file members seldom, if ever, determine organizational priorities. (Rothenberg 1992). Despite this lack of control over decision-making, members remain committed to ideological groups because of their stated purposes (Clark and Wilson 1961, 156). In fact, because they join groups based on goals, members of ideologically based organizations are more likely to influence leadership, and priorities, than members of groups in which members receive professional or economic benefits (Clark and Wilson 1961; Moe 1980; Wilson 1995 [1973]).

Additionally, existing scholarship has established the importance of some types of organizational members to group goals. Organizational leaders will pay attention to the preferences of large contributors because of the size of their contributions and the potential of their withholding donations due to disagreements with group goals. In fact, small donors perceive that their contributions are critical to the organization, sometimes mistakenly, and are therefore more likely to make their contributions dependent on group goals (Moe 1980, 80). In addition to monetary contributions to the organization, smaller contributors may also affect group goals through their service to the organization and coordination through subgroups. Economically smaller members may form subgroups, and therefore may influence organizational policy—the power of the collective will be more influential in the organization than the sum of uncoordinated smaller members (87).[7]

A member's influence on organizational priorities may be determined by his or her overall usefulness to the group. In his in-depth case study, Rothenberg finds that Common Cause's leadership set the organization's goals according to the agenda established by the activist members. Within the organization, activist members are defined as those who are critical for grassroots mobilization, are large monetary and service contributors, and have a strong ability and desire to learn and flexibly adjust their preferences based on which goals are politically, and organizationally, feasible (Rothenberg 1992, 179). According to Rothenberg's findings, such activist members set the agenda for which goals the group may pursue, leadership determines which goals will be pursued based on this agenda, and the rank and file membership have the power to veto decisions made by the leadership (181).[8]

From the literature, we know that purposive organizations are particularly concerned with keeping their members happy. Groups need their members to survive financially, but also to achieve their goals. As Roy Wilkins's quote at the beginning of the chapter illustrates, leaders of purposive organizations are aware that their membership numbers largely determine their reputation among policy-makers, as well as opportunities for funding from other sources, such as foundations. Because of such concerns, decision-makers set priorities with one eye toward how such decisions will affect the perception of the organization by its membership. Throughout the civil rights movement, some organizations struggled with how to maintain their relevance to their membership. As the goals of the movement became increasingly radicalized, established groups such as NAACP and NUL considered how to respond to the changing composition and needs of their constituencies.[9] The question then becomes, how does an organization decide which issues are important to the people, or groups of people, it claims to represent?

In the remainder of this chapter, I argue that an organization determines its priorities based on factors that are both internal and external to the organization. Specifically, I find that an organization's priorities are affected by changes in its issue niche and in the external political environment; an organization's response to such changes will be determined by its structure. My findings differ from existing literature because I do not examine internal and external factors in isolation. Rather, my reliance on each organization's archives facilitates an understanding of the interactions among factors, and their effect on organizational priorities.

The Influence of Internal Factors on Priorities

National political organizations often struggle to retain their connections to the people they represent. As groups grow, it is easy to lose contact with members and local leadership working to achieve the organization's goals (Michels 1949; Hrebenar and Scott 1982). Success in national politics sometimes requires the abandonment of grassroots tactics, such as protest organizing at the local level, in exchange for traditional tactics, such as legislative lobbying. This trade-off is unproblematic for most interest groups, which are willing to trade their grassroots connections for national exposure. However, distance from the masses is not always beneficial for constituent-based organizations, which must be concerned with the image they portray to their supporters (Truman 1960 [1951], 138; Knoke 1990, 11–12; Wilson 1973 [1995], 239).

Whether an organization relies on grassroots organizing, or inside-the-beltway lobbying, it is required to be concerned with maintaining its membership numbers—either to show up for a protest, or to be reported in a letter to Congress.[10] However, a group that regularly mobilizes its grassroots is more likely to be influenced by the concerns of local leadership, and perhaps membership (Kollman 1998; Goldstein 1999; Walker 1991). Consistent reliance on the strategy of mobilizing constituents for political action requires that a national organization coordinate with local groups, and be in close contact with local leadership to plan effective actions. Additionally, a reliance on this strategy requires that the national organization pay attention to the interests and opinion of local constituents.

Because of their concern with maintaining their connections with their local constituents, I expect national organizations to respond to calls for programming from the local level. However, I also expect that organizations' responses vary based on their internal structures. A national organization that ostensibly controls the programming of its affiliates, such as the NAACP, will be influenced by activities at the local level. However, because the national office is constitutionally responsible for determining the priorities of local branches, this influence may not come from the local offices themselves. Instead, the national office will be influenced by the activities of other organizations in the field, like SNCC, that are mobilizing people that both groups consider to be part of their constituencies (Clark and Wilson 1961; Wilson 1973 [1995]; Gray and Lowery 1996).[11] To maintain its membership, political strength, and preeminence within its issue niche, an organization will work to prevent the loss of its constituency, or potential constituency, to other organizations with similar missions.

For large organizations with autonomous affiliates, such as CORE, NUL, and SCLC, affiliate activities may determine national priorities because the national office seeks to retain relevance to its chapters. In such organizations with federated structures, the national office does not pursue its own priorities, but rather exists to coordinate, and perhaps guide, local chapter programming. If the national office does not maintain a cooperative relationship with its local chapters, the chapters are able to pursue their own priorities without regard to the national organization, stripping the national office of its purpose. In such federated groups, I expect that the national office will shape its priorities according to those of the local offices.

Civil rights organizations varied in their anti-poverty activities, but all acknowledged the reality of the disproportionate numbers of African Americans living in poverty after the legislative victories of the mid-1960s. Calls for national-level anti-poverty activity primarily came from organizations at the local level, or within national organizations that focused on grassroots organizing during the civil rights movement (Carson 1995; Peake 1987). I analyze organizational charts, affiliate directives, internal communications, funding of affiliates and chapters, and organizational histories to determine the national office's direction of local offices. For example, the NUL devoted itself to restructuring its relationship with its affiliates beginning in the early 1960s. As I detail in Chapter 5, internal memos at the national level provide insight into the national office's commitment to this change, and the purpose of the increasing national oversight of affiliate activities. Public documents, such as annual reports, provide insight into whether the national office took responsibility for local programming, and which programming the national office oversaw.

The Influence of External Variables on Interest Group Priorities

An examination of a national office's relationship with its local branches and other local organizations will shed light on how it interacts with, and perceives the preferences of, its membership or constituency. However, imagining that only internal factors affect priorities is unrealistic—an organization does not exist in a bubble, disconnected from other groups or the political world. Factors external to the organization, such as the activities of other groups with similar missions, or the group's relationship with political elites, will contribute to its assessment of the priorities it must pursue to maintain its membership, and its preeminence within its issue niche.

Relations Among Organizations in the Same Issue Niche

According to pluralist theory, varying political interests gain representation because of group competition for membership. Scholars have assessed the levels of competition among organizations, how this competition operates in the political system, and which interests benefit from the rivalries among groups.[12] In their analysis of incentive systems, Clark and Wilson (1961) argue that a group faces varying levels of competition from rival organizations based on the types of incentives it offers to its members. To maintain membership, and attract contributions, a purposive organization will often specialize in particular policy areas or tactics to achieve its goals. Clark and Wilson argue, however, that the increasing number of interest groups makes such autonomy difficult to maintain. As the number of groups proliferate, it is particularly difficult for organizations to maintain their areas of specialization. Competition increases if multiple organizations are addressing the same ends, and differences among organizations become less clear to membership. According to pluralist theory, this competition among groups insures that multiple interests within the system gain representation.[13] Threats to an organization's autonomy from other groups may cause a group leader to respond by shifting goals to please the highest number of members, or potential members (Clark and Wilson 1961; Wilson 1973 [1995]; Gray and Lowery 1996).

Scholars have also argued that competition within an organization may lead to a shift in priorities. One of the primary goals of an organization's leadership is to prevent the formation of subgroups within the organization that may lead to rival groups (Salisbury 1969, 29). Moe argues that if a leader is required to focus on the specific needs of rival groups, she or he has less time to devote to the needs of the organization's general membership. The effect then becomes circular—the general membership becomes displeased because it feels neglected by the organization's leadership, and therefore forms subgroups that plan to secede from the original organization (Moe 1980, 133–37). Therefore, through the threat of rival leadership, subgroups are able to gain the attention of organizational leaders, even if their issues are not regarded as pertinent to the interests of the entire membership (140).

Moe's (1980) analysis of subgroups within organizations, and Clark and Wilson's analysis of incentive systems, may be applied to competitive organizations within issue niches. If several organizations compose a niche, relations can be harmonious as long as groups are not required to compete over membership. This may be possible if groups carve out their own priorities within each niche, or approach the same social problem with differing tactics. Even the threat of competition from groups with similar missions causes organizations to protect their role within the issue niche. A group may also avoid competition by shifting its focus within its overall mission, or focusing on a different aspect of its "identity" (Heaney 2004). Strolovitch (2007) finds that such "niche behavior" among advocacy groups suppresses activity on behalf of disadvantaged subpopulations. Because they often do not "belong" to one interest niche, intersectional issues provide an opportunity for redefinitions of organizational identity (109). However, within a group of organizations that arguably share a defined constituency, such as civil rights groups, perceived competition for membership may be inevitable, regardless of the various options for organizational focus and strategy.[14] Furthermore, if one organization within the niche approaches general goals from a new perspective, one that appeals to a broad base of membership, competition to maintain membership may require shifts in organizations' goals and priorities toward those of the rival organization. Because it is important for a group to maintain its membership, and therefore its preeminence within its issue niche, competition will force organizations to adjust their goals to appeal to the broadest component of their constituency.

As other scholars have documented, civil rights groups cooperated as a movement with common goals, and also competed with each other for the support of potential constituencies throughout the 1960s (Garrow 1986; Zald and Garner 1987; Peake 1987; Morris 1984). What is less established, however, are the implications of these relationships on group priorities. My method of analysis offers a unique opportunity to examine intergroup relations and the effect of those relations within organizations. Because I am analyzing the archives of five of the most prominent organizations within an issue niche, I am able to understand how relations among the groups affect internal decision-making and priority-setting.

I rely on internal memoranda, and documents pertaining to coalition work, to analyze the relations among groups, and the effect of these relations on group goals. Internal memos sometimes made the organizational concern with competition explicit:

> Today there are competitive organizations in the field. . . . They feel that if they can carve out a role for themselves and thus diminish the strength and agility of the larger civil rights organizations in the field, that they will be able to corner the civil rights market and take control of it.[15]

For other organizations, internal memos were not so explicit. For example, a group's public statements about its relevance to the civil rights struggle may speak to the influence of intergroup competition on its goals.

The Influence of Political Elites on Organizational Priorities

When organizations are determining the policy priorities they will pursue, it seems intuitive that leadership would consider the response of policymakers. Without the support of lawmakers, the organization's goals may be doomed from the start. Resource mobilization theorists have argued that groups benefit from elite support in terms of policy success, and the ability to raise money (McCarthy and Zald 1973). However, scholars have found that it is not always in an organization's best interest to achieve the support of political elites. In fact, the influence of policy elites on an organization's priorities varies based on a group's structure.

Within social movements, scholars have found that the relationship between movement organizations and political actors is complex. McAdam (1982) argues that in movements composed of people who are excluded from the political system, and who engage in tactics meant to fundamentally alter the existing system, elite support may actually harm the movement. As McAdam argues, organizations such as SNCC may lose legitimacy in the eyes of its constituency if it works too closely with political elites, or relies on funding that is contingent on elite support. On the other hand, other organizations within the same movement, such as the NUL, may be quite concerned with elite support of its goals, because it relies on government contract support for funding.

To assess the impact of political elites on the goals of civil rights organizations, I examine evidence of a relationship between each organization and political parties, the president, and Congress. Testimonies at congressional hearings and party committee conventions, meetings with

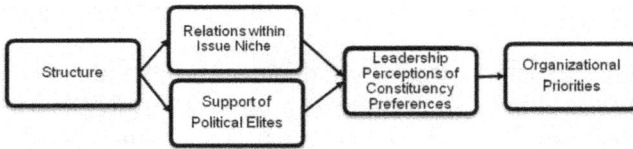

Figure 2.1. Factors determining organizational priorities.

committee staff, speeches by committee representatives at the organizations' conventions, and civil rights leaders' participation in Democratic and Republican Caucuses all indicate each organization's relationship with political elites. However, these formal measures of relations between parties and organizations may not capture the full story of relations among elites and organizations. Only the NAACP and the NUL testified before Congress concerning anti-poverty policy during the 1960s and 1970s.[17] It would be inaccurate to conclude that only the NAACP and the NUL had relationships with elites that might have influenced their priorities. Therefore, I also examine less formal communications between civil rights organizations and political elites, such as meetings with White House and administrative staff and communications with congressional staff. These communications indicate the level of attention paid by elites to organizational priorities, as well as the organization's attention to the opinions of elites.

Assessing Influences on Organizational Goals

Central to my understanding of the factors determinant of organizational goals is an organization's attention to its membership. My theory falls in line with those who argue for the importance of internal processes for organizational decision making (Moe 1980; Rothenberg 1992; Wilson 1995 [1973]). I also find external factors to be determinative of priorities, both through their effects on internal operations of organizations, and as constraints on organizational behavior (Walker 1991; Gray and Lowery 1996; March and Olsen 1989). However, as Figure 2.1 reflects, I do not anticipate that either internal or external factors alone determine organizational priorities—the interaction of such factors lead to shifts in goals. As I demonstrate in the following chapters, my findings indicate that the effect of external factors on organizational priorities varies based on the group's internal structure.

In the next chapter, I begin my analysis of the civil rights activities concerning poverty policy during the 1960s. In the 1960s, some civil rights organizations chose to respond to the War on Poverty with protests and lobbying, and placed increasing importance on mobilizing low-income African Americans. Other groups lobbied Congress and mobilized local branches to work to implement the EOA. The groups varied in their levels of commitment to the War on Poverty, facilitating assessments of the varieties of factors leading to priority shifts within organizations.

Chapter 3

Civil Rights Organizations and the War on Poverty

> Despite passage of the most sweeping Federal legislation since Reconstruction, Negro citizens may wake up one morning to find themselves with a mouthful of civil rights and an empty dinner table, living in a hovel.
> —Whitney Young, Director, National Urban League, 1964

Because of the persisting relationship between race and poverty, civil rights organizations have advocated on behalf of low-income African Americans throughout their histories. Civil rights organizations vary in their founding level of commitment to poverty, and to economic issues in general. One of the NUL's founding missions was to provide job training for African Americans; SNCC's founding statement indicated the effects of poverty on African Americans. In fact, each civil rights organization made some mention of economic inequity in their mission statements. However, as will be demonstrated in this chapter, each organization's implementation of their missions varied. For some groups, such as SNCC and CORE, poverty became an increasingly critical issue as activists in the field were confronted with the effects of poverty on voter registration in the South. Increasing attention to the effects of poverty by national organizations pushed the issue onto the national stage, and required responses from each organization within the civil rights issue niche.

In this and the next chapter, I consider the level of attention that the NUL, NAACP, CORE, SCLC, and SNCC devoted to anti-poverty policy during the 1960s and 1970s. In this chapter, I assess each group's attention to anti-poverty policy leading up to, and concerning, the Economic Opportunity Act of 1964. I also examine CORE, SNCC, and SCLC anti-poverty activities during the late 1960s. In the next chapter, I assess the NAACP's and NUL anti-poverty activities during the late 1960s and concerning the Family Assistance Plan in the early 1970s. This over-time comparison of activities and priority levels allows me to establish the levels of attention that organizations devoted to advocacy on behalf of the poor. It is shifts in these levels that I explain in the remainder of this book.

Responses to the Crisis in Public Welfare (1960–1968)

Because of the increasing costs of public assistance policies during the 1950s, federal and state policymakers turned their attention to welfare provision in the early 1960s. State-led changes to the Aid to Dependent Children programs during 1960 and 1961 generally involved cuts in benefits, work requirements, and measures that restricted welfare receipt for unwed mothers. Responding to such measures in the states, Congress explicitly changed AFDC rules to encourage welfare mothers to work, and included incentives such as training and social services designed to increase their employability (Abramovitz 2000, 79). President Kennedy prioritized such reforms to the Social Security system in his first address to Congress.[1]

Kennedy's Amendments implemented significant changes to the public welfare system; in 1964 the system faced its greatest overhaul since the New Deal. On August 20, 1964, Congress passed the EOA, which established anti-poverty policy as a priority of the Johnson administration. With the support of labor, business, and advocacy groups, the EOA was drafted and passed without fervent opposition. Although this support would be short-lived—for example, labor groups eventually opposed particular nondiscrimination policies implemented by the newly created Office of Economic Opportunity—passage of the legislation occurred with widespread support.[2]

The purpose of the EOA was to alleviate poverty in urban centers, particularly among African Americans, as well as rural poverty. The Act was considered unique by policy-makers, as well as advocacy groups, because of its emphasis on the involvement of the poor through Title II, which included the creation of the OEO, and the legislation's "maximum feasible participation" clause. The Title's overall principle was that the poor should participate in the newly established local anti-poverty agencies, Community Action Programs (CAPs) (Axinn and Stern, 2001, 247). Although funded by the federal government, each CAP would be run by local agencies and nonprofit organizations, opening the door to possible interest group participation in the implementation of the EOA (Jackson 1993, 419).

After the passage and initial implementation of the Act, the War on Poverty immediately faced opposition and attempts to cut funding and programming. Both liberals and conservatives questioned whether a government bureaucracy could be effective in combating poverty. *The Negro Family: The Case for National Action*, or the Moynihan Report, was released in by the U.S. Department of Labor in March 1965, and pointed to weaknesses in the African American family structure as road-blocks to economic equality. According to the Report, black women were too strong within the African American family structure, and pre-vented black men from gaining and exerting authority. The Report gained widespread attention, and support varied among civil rights groups. George Wiley of CORE was outspoken in his critiques of the Report and its over-reliance on behavior as an explanation of poverty. Other leaders, such as Martin Luther King, Jr., Roy Wilkins, and Whitney Young endorsed the Report.[3] Despite these differences among groups, no civil rights organization shaped its policy response to the War on Poverty in terms of the Moynihan Report; instead groups focused on addressing the structural bases for inequality. However, organizations did address perverse incentives within the welfare program, such as the inability for a woman to receive aid if she lived with a man. Such policy created a disincentive for families to stay together, according to the Moy-nihan Report and civil rights organizations.[4]

As the number of women and children receiving AFDC increased after the passage of the EOA, critics pointed to policy change as con-tributing to family instability, reflecting the concerns stated in the Moynihan Report (Abramovitz 2000, 81). In 1967, Congress passed the amendments to the EOA. Although the amendments were initially pro-posed by the Johnson administration to increase Aid to Families with Dependent Children (AFDC) benefits, the bill that came out of the House Ways and Means Committee cut benefits, froze program expan-sion, and introduced work requirements for single mothers (Noble 1997, 97).

The NAACP, NUL, CORE, SCLC, and SNCC were all active concern-ing anti-poverty policy during the 1960s. However, the groups varied in their attention to the issue. Some groups prioritized advocacy on behalf of the poor before the War on Poverty, while others rarely addressed welfare policy. Across organizations, the civil rights advocacy that did occur was focused on demanding nondiscriminatory implementation of welfare rules in the states. Once the federal government waged the War on Poverty, the NAACP, NUL, and SNCC considered anti-poverty to be

Table 3.1. Organizational Positions on Economic Opportunity Act

Organization	Position on EOA (War on Poverty)
NAACP	• Support of EOA • Working toward nondiscriminatory implementation and engagement of poor.
NUL	• Strong support of EOA • Actively engaged with legislative drafting • Claims credit for EOA provisions that were included in League Domestic Marshall Plan
CORE	• No national office position on EOA • Concerned about nondiscriminatory implementation, but also with federal government approach to poverty alleviation
SCLC	• No position taken on EOA • Concerned with nondiscriminatory implementation
SNCC	• Strong opposition to federal government approach to poverty alleviation

a programming priority. The organizations varied in their approach to poverty—the NAACP and NUL worked to support the War on Poverty, while SNCC remained highly critical of the federal government's programs. CORE and the SCLC did not devote organizational attention to anti-poverty policy until the War on Poverty programs came under attack during the late 1960s. Table 3.1 summarizes the variety in positions on the EOA across organizations.

In the next section, I examine each group's advocacy on behalf of the poor during the 1960s and establish the level of priority each organization gave to anti-poverty policy.

The NAACP Response to Anti-Poverty Programs

Throughout the early and mid-1960s, the NAACP was primarily focused on issues of nondiscrimination, planning the 1963 March on Washington, passage and implementation of the Civil Rights Act of 1964 and the Voting Rights Act of 1965, the passage of the twenty fourth amendment making poll taxes unconstitutional, in addition to numerous court cases in the states and at the federal level.[5] Throughout its history the NAACP has had a reputation for elitism and a lack of concern with the plight of low-income African Americans. By the mid-1950s, the organization addressed issues confronting African American workers primarily through policy advocacy, and not litigation strategy, which became largely confined to cases involving nondiscrimination and desegregation (Frymer 2008; Goluboff 2007).

As Table 3.2 illustrates, NAACP attention to public assistance policies was scant until 1964 and 1965. Although the organization offered rhetoric concerning poverty during the early 1960s, it did not engage in activities that brought the issue to the attention of its membership or policymakers. During the War on Poverty, on the other hand, the NAACP devoted significant financial resources to the program, and mobilized its membership and branches to be active in its implementation. As poverty issues became increasingly important within the civil rights movement of during the early 1960s, the NAACP struggled with whether and how it would address the interests of low-income African Americans. My measurements of priority reflect this change: the NAACP increased its involvement from 8 percent of possible anti-poverty activities in the early 1960s, to 57 percent of possible activities in 1964 and 1965.

NAACP Anti-Poverty Activities (1960–1963)

NAACP attention to public assistance policies was limited until 1964 and 1965; however, the organization sporadically offered critiques of the U.S. welfare system. Beginning in 1961, the Board passed resolutions specifically addressing public welfare, and the inequitable disbursement of welfare benefits between African Americans and whites. The organization's overall approach was to combat implementation of state welfare laws that discriminated against African Americans, and which were generally dehumanizing to eligible mothers and their children. In both 1961 and 1962, a convention resolution specifically addressed attempts by numerous states to deny benefits to eligible recipients based on residency requirements, and to disparage the character of welfare recipients, particularly women accused to intentionally having additional children to increase their welfare payments:

> Throughout the country there is a growing campaign . . . to discredit the principle of humane and efficient public assistance to persons unable to maintain themselves. This has taken the form of efforts to malign newcomers by charging, without basis in fact, that they have deliberately migrated to urban areas in order to seek welfare and other public assistance and of claims that many women are taking advantage of the ADC program through illegitimacy to increase their benefits and that many able-bodied reject employment in favor of public assistance. . . . We call on our branches and state conferences to investigate all instances of denial of public assistance where such denial is racially motivated and to take affirmative action through appropriate statements, protests and other means to insure

Table 3.2. NAACP Prioritization of Anti-Poverty Policy, 1960–1965

Organizational activities	Pre-EOA (1960–1963)	Immediate response to EOA (1964–1965)
Low-priority indicators (1 point each)		
• Position taken on issue (statement, convention, resolution)	X	X
Mid-level priority indicators (2 points each)		
• Staff, or organizational committee, assigned to issue as one of several, or only, assignments		X
• Internal evidence of funding for activities concerning issue		
• Communications to policy-makers about issue (testimonies before Congress or parties, position letters)		X
• Public speeches or statements by staff/ leadership about issue		X
• National office directs local branches/ affiliates to be active on issue	X	X
• Mailings to membership about issue		
High-level priority indicators (3 points each)		
• Fundraising with membership about issue		
• Mobilization of membership for actions about issue		
• Consultation with policy-makers about issue (legislative drafting, implementation)		X
• National office offers workshops/training for local branches/affiliates on issue		X
• Internal discussions, as reflected in meeting minutes and transcripts, indicate issue as priority		X
• Organizational documents name the issue as a priority (resolutions, annual reports, org. publications)		X
• Organizational restructuring to address issue (overall restructuring, creation of new department)		
• Organization offers own plan concerning issue		
No evidence of priority		
• Absence of any evidence of issue as priority		
*Priority level**	8%	57%

*Priority level determined by organization activities as percentage of total possible activities. NAACP activities during early 1960s totaled 3 of 37 possible points, an 8% priority score; War on Poverty period totaled 22 of 37 possible points, a 57% priority score.

that the rights of innocent children and all other necessitous persons are protected.[6]

In 1962, the Board passed a resolution linking economic and social factors to the reasons why a disproportionate number of African Americans were eligible to receive welfare benefits, and supporting benefit provision to children with a father in the home. Such a provision would help to eradicate the negative portrayal of African American women recipients, who were being portrayed as taking advantage of the system.[7]

> The high proportion of Negro families receiving such assistance in many communities is used to reflect discredit upon the race of these recipients . . . economic and social factors, such as continued higher levels of unemployment among Negroes, should be pointed up as contributing to this unfortunate situation . . . since gainful employment is too often denied the Negro male, [we urge that] there be a renewal of the temporary provision allowing assistance to dependent children even if an employable male is in the home, when the unemployment is through no fault of his own.[8]

During the 1962 convention, the organization asked branches "to investigate all denials of public assistance where racially motivated and to take affirmative action through issuance of appropriate statements, protests and other means to insure protection of rights of innocent children and other necessitous persons."[9]

The national office itself was not active concerning welfare reform or welfare legislation during the early 1960s. Although directives concerning discrimination by state welfare agencies were issued to branches and resolutions stating the organization's positions were passed at conventions, there is no evidence that the national office played a role in the passage of President Kennedy's public assistance amendments of 1962.

The NAACP Response to the War on Poverty

As Table 3.2 illustrates, the NAACP increased its activities during 1964 and 1965 to a mid-level of priority. After President Johnson presented the War on Poverty in his State of the Union Address, the NAACP issued a statement supporting the president's proposed plans:

> Poverty, disease, war and racial inequities are the enemies against which [Johnson] seeks a national mobilization of our total resources, material and spiritual. His moving challenge deserves to be met with prompt Congressional action and with the cooperation of all citizens in their everyday pursuits.[10]

The NAACP statement indicates the national office's support for federal action on issues of poverty; the organization had never before issued such a statement concerning public assistance legislation.

In September 1964, at its first meeting since the EOA's passage, the Board voted to appoint a Special Committee to study the Anti-Poverty Act, and to present formal guidelines for branches to follow: "As to the Anti-Poverty Act, we must devise ways of working on the community level. . . . We must study it and devise ways and means of getting in on the ground floor, on the local level."[11] The next month, the Special Committee reported that it was preparing a memorandum outlining the Anti-Poverty Act for the branches, and indicating the most appropriate areas for NAACP involvement.[12] By this time, the national office had already received word that branches were "moving rapidly ahead to implement [EOA] programs" from the organization's regional offices.[13] The November issue of *The Crisis*, the NAACP newsletter, named the implementation of the EOA as the organization's top priority, and the branches' activities were reported.[14] Shortly after the national office named the anti-poverty legislation as its top priority, Herbert Hill, Labor Secretary and a member of the Special Committee, presented his proposal for NAACP involvement in the anti-poverty programs: he proposed that "the NAACP become the basic coordinating agency in the Negro community for initiating, negotiating, and operating programs developed under the authority of the Economic Opportunity Act of 1964."[15]

In 1965, the NAACP passed its most detailed, and policy-based, resolution concerning the organization's welfare-related activities.

> The NAACP recognizes . . . the EOA as a great challenge to the American people and an equally great opportunity for the American Negro and all other minorities . . . We believe the NAACP can make a significant contribution to the War on Poverty and urge our national officers, branches, and members to pursue constructive and aggressive courses of action.[16]

Although national and local staff generally recognized the importance of placing immediate priority on the War on Poverty, some affiliates were ill-equipped to make such a transition. In early 1965, Hill wrote to Roy Wilkins explaining that branches would require significant help from the national office to be able to participate in local anti-poverty programs effectively. "Because the NAACP has traditionally eschewed social work approaches . . . there will be a reluctance as already indicated, on the part of government agencies to enter into contractual agreements with the NAACP." Therefore, Hill stated that branches would need "extensive intervention" by the national office, and that this help could not be limited to memos.[17] The Board voted to create a manual for the branches to guide them in their participation in the anti-poverty programs at the local level. Branches were to seek representation on local CAP planning boards, and to demand representative participation of African Americans throughout the phases of the poverty program.[18] The organization's 1965 annual report highlighted the anti-poverty activities of numerous branches and State Conferences.[19] Although the organization's focus on poverty was new as compared to the early 1960s, the NAACP retained its themes of nondiscriminatory implementation and equal access to welfare benefits.

Although Wilkins gave support to the findings of the Moynihan report, the NAACP did not focus its policy advocacy on behavioral change among African Americans, and instead increased its advocacy based on its understanding of the structural bases of poverty. By 1965, the NAACP's activities reflected a commitment to rely on the federal government to provide aid for those who were ineligible to receive contributory benefits. The national office mobilized its branches, met with policymakers, and named the War on Poverty as an organizational priority after the passage of the EOA.

NUL Attention to Anti-Poverty Policy During the 1960s

Prior to the passage of the EOA, the NUL considered anti-poverty policy to be a priority. In fact, the NUL and its allies on the Hill and in the White House considered the NUL "Domestic Marshall Plan," drafted in 1963, to be an inspiration for President Johnson's War on Poverty, and a precursor to the EOA.[20] Passed by the 1963 Annual Conference, the Domestic Marshall Plan included public welfare provisions, calling for coverage of unemployed parents in the ADC program, job training to increase the eventual employability of recipients, and funding for child care facilities.[21] The League was also actively engaged in planning the 1963 March on Washington, and remained committed to its goals of ensuring employment, job throughout the early and mid-1960s (Dickerson 1998).

After President Johnson declared war on poverty during his 1964 State of the Union address, Whitney Young, executive director, saw the possibility for the NUL to expand its programming activities substantially. Johnson's War on Poverty did not create the NUL's interest in antipoverty policy—the organization had consistently been concerned with social welfare policy generally, and specifically with public assistance policy. However, the passage of the EOA, and the possibility of injecting the NUL with millions of federal dollars, caused the organization to make EOA implementation its central priority during the mid- to late 1960s. Table 3.3 illustrates this shift—the NUL participated in 59 percent of possible anti-poverty activities during the early 1960s and 100 percent during the War on Poverty.

Table 3.3. NUL Prioritization of Anti-Poverty Policy, 1960–1965

Organizational activities	Pre-EOA (1960–1963)	Immediate response to EOA (1964–1965)
Low-priority indicators (1 point each)		
• Position taken on issue (statement, convention resolution)	X	X
Mid-level priority indicators (2 points each)		
• Staff, or organizational committee, assigned to issue as one of several, or only, assignments		X
• Internal evidence of funding for activities concerning issue		X
• Communications to policy-makers about issue (testimonies before Congress or parties, position letters)	X	X
• Public speeches or statements by staff/ leadership about issue	X	X
• National office directs local branches/ affiliates to be active on issue	X	X
• Mailings to membership about issue*	N/A	N/A
High-level priority indicators (3 points each)		X
• Fundraising with membership about issue**		
• Mobilization of membership for actions about issue*	N/A	N/A
• Consultation with policy-makers about issue (legislative drafting, implementation)	X	X
• National office offers workshops/training for local branches/affiliates on issue		X
• Internal discussions, as reflected in meeting minutes and transcripts, indicate issue as priority	X	X
• Organizational documents name the issue as a priority (resolutions, annual reports, org. publications)	X	X
• Organizational restructuring to address issue (overall restructuring, creation of new department)		X
• Organization offers own plan concerning issue	X	X
No evidence of priority		
Absence of any evidence of issue as priority		
*Priority level****	59%	100%

*NUL is not a mass-membership organization; these categories do not apply.
**Indicates fundraising in terms of receiving corporate or foundation grants.
***Priority level determined by organization activities as percentage of total possible activities. NUL activities during early 1960s totaled 21 of 32 possible points, a 59% priority score; War on Poverty period totaled 32 of 32 possible points, a 100% priority score.

NUL Attention to Anti-Poverty During the Early 1960s

Before the War on Poverty, and the passage of the EOA, the League was active concerning anti-poverty policy, and considered public assistance policies to be one of its areas of focus. When Louisiana passed legislation that denied welfare benefits to unwed mothers, the national office sent a public memo to local Urban Leagues urging their response: "an event of deep national significance has aroused little or no widespread reaction . . . such public inaction is dangerous to the welfare standards of the country."[22] The national office argued that the cuts to the ADC program were racially motivated: "this wave of anti-ADC action . . . has developed from ignorance [and] calculated malice . . . used by hard-crusted reactionaries or racist agitators."[23] As additional states began to consider ADC cuts and new requirements for recipients, the national office encouraged local affiliates to take action, especially in coalition with other organizations.[24]

In 1961, the city of Newburgh, New York, attempted to impose tight restrictions on welfare recipients, including work requirements for men, benefit loss for unwed mothers having additional children, and requirements that new welfare applicants show proof of employment when they arrived in Newburgh (Abramovitz 2000, 75; Patterson 1994, 104). The NUL opposed the actions of the city council, and wrote to the state Board of Welfare in New York pointing to the similarities of Newburgh's actions and those in Louisiana the year before. In his letter, Henry Steeger, NUL president, argued that the city's statements that potential recipients were moving to Newburgh simply to receive benefits required study and empirical documentation.[25] Steeger offered the services of the NUL to the State Board to address the situation in Newburgh with "wisdom and humanity."[26] The NUL was monitoring legislation to cut benefits in numerous states, and asked affiliates to report such legislation, and their activities concerning it, to the national office.[27]

The NUL was active concerning the Kennedy administration's proposed amendments to the Social Security Act, and tracked the legislation's progress through Congress. Based on its founding mission as primarily a social service agency, the League considered advocacy for the provision of public welfare benefits to be central to its overall mission. When the House Ways and Means Committee amended the proposal with provisions, which the NUL considered punitive to recipients, the organization's Health and Welfare Department informed staff of the danger of these changes, and reminded the League: "The Urban League's stake in a constructive public welfare program is obviously high."[28] After the passage of the amendments, the NUL reported to the Department of Health, Education, and Welfare that "through memos, conferences, and field visits we are urging Urban League leadership to move ahead on stimulating implementation of the public welfare amendments at the state level."[29]

Seven months before President Johnson declared a "War on Poverty," the 1963 NUL Conference adopted a resolution on public welfare calling for affiliate activities, and defining the welfare provisions with which the organization should be particularly concerned:

> [Urban League Boards] should take decisive action in examining and ana-
> lyzing the public welfare laws of their states and to improve and strengthen
> them in order to take advantage of the Federal public welfare pro-
> visions; . . . the Urban League [should] give emphasis to these particular
> provisions in the amendments: coverage of unemployed parent in ADC
> programs; community work training programs; day care facilities.[30]

In addition to a focus on these policy provisions, the NUL was concerned with African American representation in the public welfare bureaucracy. The League worked to recruit blacks to leadership positions in welfare departments at the local, state, and national levels.[31]

The NUL was unique among civil rights organizations because of its focus on poverty in the early 1960s and because of its overall prioritization of public assistance policy before the passage of the EOA. As Table 3.2 illustrates, the NUL's attention to anti-poverty policy during the early 1960s reflects a mid-level of priority.

The NUL Role in the War on Poverty (1964–1966)

President Johnson introduced the EOA on March 16, 1964 in a special message to Congress. After Johnson introduced the Act, Whitney Young, executive director, wrote to him and indicated the NUL commitment to the implementation of the EOA programs: "Through our Regional Offices and our 65 affiliates and in urban centers throughout the country, it will be possible for the League to contribute importantly toward overcoming the national problem of poverty."[32] In his message to Johnson, Young promised the commitment of the NUL at the national, regional, and local levels. Reflecting this commitment, the national office announced its plans for a major reorganization and expansion programs "to combat poverty and despair among Negroes" in April 1964.[33] Additional regional offices and local branches were founded, and the structure of the organization was changed to give more authority to regional directors, allowing for easy coordination with the proposed OEO. The NUL's reorganization, and the national office's focus on mobilizing its affiliates concerning the War on Poverty, is reflected in the organization's high level of participation in anti-poverty activities during 1964 and 1965.[34]

The War on Poverty presented an opportunity for NUL to receive government funding to carry out existing priorities. The Johnson administration promised to guide the NUL as it drafted its War on Poverty grant proposals.[35] Additionally, the NUL counted on its commitment to the administration to secure funding:

> the time spent with Mr. Shriver in drawing up the bill and stepping up the program . . . and the fact that five program staff people are presently in Washington for meetings with top staff of the program . . . make certain that NUL moves in the right direction to secure grants under this program . . . even if a local Urban League does not receive money directly.[36]

In May 1964, the national office held a War on Poverty Workshop for Urban League affiliate executive directors and regional directors. Officials informed affiliates that they should be prepared to become involved with the implementation of the EOA by "identifying needs of the Negro in . . . local communities" and "conduct[ing] an inventory of the policies and practices of public and private welfare agencies, institutions . . . serving the needy."[37] The national office sent local affiliates specific guidelines concerning the proposed CAPs, how they would be structured, and how local Urban Leagues could best position themselves to participate in the programs.[38] After this conference, and after receiving input from the League's affiliates, the national office's Program staff voted to "give . . . priority to the War on Poverty" and to offer Sargent Shriver, Director of the OEO, use of Urban League personnel on a part-time basis.[39]

The League prioritization of the War on Poverty was again made explicit at its 1964 conference: delegates were urged mobilize citizen participation in the organization's four areas of prime concern: "1) the Anti-Poverty War; 2) the new Civil Rights Act; 3) Urban riots; 4) Nonpartisan voter education."[40] Regional directors were informed of their duties concerning implementation of the War on Poverty—the national office would assess the effectiveness of local Leagues based on their participation on anti-poverty boards:

> The regional directors . . . are charged to see that local Urban Leagues make efforts to form cooperative groups to secure anti-poverty program commitments or get on the boards of existing groups. The National office will be checking . . . to see that each Urban League is involved in the anti-poverty effort and will assess the skill of local Urban League executives on the basis of such activity.[41]

The national office was particularly concerned with local activities because EOA implementation would be concentrated at the local level.

Regional staff were asked to collect information from local affiliates about the types of existing welfare programming in their cities, with the hope of inciting the affiliates to take action in the implementation of the anti-poverty programs. National staff encouraged local affiliates to work with mayors and other community leaders to develop implementation plans for the War on Poverty, and to take the lead on such planning if necessary.[42]

Delegates at the 1964 conference passed two resolutions concerning anti-poverty policy and the president's proposed War on Poverty—one included policy recommendations, and the other concerned NUL involvement with the war. These resolutions would guide the national office in its positions and priorities for the coming year. NUL delegates voted in support of indexing public assistance payments to inflation. Opposing federal penalties for marriage, the delegates voted in support of allowing payments to go to families with an unemployed father in the home. The national conference also voted to "establish special national staff . . . and regional workers for the primary purpose of programming and coordinating the Urban League's attack on poverty."[43] Three weeks after the conference, Congress passed the EOA. By that time, the War on Poverty was undoubtedly the organization's top priority, and the NUL was in a position to receive substantial federal government funding for anti-poverty programming.

Immediately after the passage of the EOA, the NUL began planning its Community Action Assembly to discuss the implementation of the War on Poverty. The NUL invited administration officials and more than three hundred civil rights leaders to Washington, D.C., in December 1964 to discuss how to use the anti-poverty and civil rights legislation to combat poverty and discrimination: "The meeting will examine thoroughly the provisions under the Federal Government's anti-poverty program and evaluate methods of implementing the Federal civil rights bill."[44] The Johnson administration participated in the Assembly: the president; Sargent Shriver, director of the OEO; Anthony J. Celebrezze, Secretary of Health, Education and Welfare; and W. Willard Wirtz, Secretary of Labor, addressed the participants.[45]

After the Community Action Assembly, the NUL began planning numerous regional and state poverty workshops to "stimulate grass roots participation in the implementation of the EOA."[46] In addition to increasing community activity concerning the EOA, the Southern Regional Office touted the workshops as opportunities for the community to have contact with government officials, and to gain assurances that EOA programs would primarily serve the poor.[47] The NUL also hoped that the workshops would change its elitist reputation. The national office worried that if it did not expand its contact with low-income African Americans, the OEO would not consider the NUL an appropriate recipient of War on Poverty grants.[48]

The Johnson administration continued to recognize the NUL's commitment to the War on Poverty, and to rely on the organization for advice. Beginning in 1965, Whitney Young became a member of the Office of Economic Opportunity's Advisory Committee.[49] At the 55th Annual Conference in 1965, Young introduced the League's "Agenda for the Future"—a 10-point program to remedy the effects of poverty.[50] Delegates at the convention passed a lengthy resolution concerning public assistance.

> the Public Assistance programs in nearly all states are inadequate to meet the needs of those who must depend upon them because of the low level of assistance payments, the imposition of residence requirements . . . gaps in the programs which leave many needy people without an available program of aid, and the application of eligibility requirements unrelated to the needs of the applicant. . . . the US Congress [is] requested to amend the Social Security Act to provide a more adequate public assistance program to meet the needs of those who must depend upon such assistance.[51]

The Resolution went on to request that Congress redefine eligibility to be determined solely based on need, establish a federally mandated benefit floor, improve the social services offered to recipients, and to remove requirements that otherwise qualified people and families have residences to receive benefits.[52] This Resolution reflects the League's overall commitment to federal anti-poverty programming and nondiscrimination in the implementation of that programming.

The NUL commitment to alleviating poverty, and to offering social services to the poor, was established upon the organization's founding. Once the federal government began to consider a widespread anti-poverty program, the NUL considered its involvement necessary to insure nondiscriminatory implementation of programs. The League advised the Johnson Administration throughout the drafting of the legislation, and maintained its proprietary relationship with the War on Programs throughout the mid-1960s. Similar to the NAACP, the League strongly maintained its policy focus on alleviating the structural bases of poverty, and did not emphasize behavioral change among African Americans. However, unlike other civil rights organizations, the NUL considered the War on Poverty to be its central priority—its reorganization, directions to local office, relations with policymakers, and certainly its rhetoric, reflected this commitment.

CORE Anti-Poverty Activities During the 1960s

Beginning in the early 1960s, CORE actively sought to expand its constituency beyond the middle and upper classes, and to rid itself of its intellectual and elite reputation. Amid CORE's grassroots organizing, including the coordination of the 1961 Freedom Ride, the national office encouraged chapters to expand their activities to include the poor. After the Freedom Ride, CORE focused less attention on desegregation in public accommodations, and emphasized access to housing, job nondiscrimination, and voter registration in its programming (Meier and Rudwick 1975 [1973]). Although the organization did not advocate on behalf of low-income African Americans during the early 1960s, CORE's emphasis on expanding its constituency set the stage for increasing attention to the poor during the late 1960s. As Table 3.4 indicates, CORE increased its attention to anti-poverty during the mid-1960s, but continued to give such activities low priority. Nonetheless, the organization did increase its advocacy on behalf of the poor as compared to its activities during the early 1960s. Between 1960 and 1963, CORE performed only 5 percent of possible anti-poverty activities; during 1964 and 1965, the organization's priority score increased to 27 percent. It was not until the late 1960s that CORE placed a high level of priority on anti-poverty policy. Between 1966 and 1968, CORE was involved in 68 percent of possible anti-poverty activities.

CORE Concern with Welfare Policy During the Early 1960s

At CORE's 1962 convention, director James Farmer emphasized the need to expand the organization's recruitment efforts to include low-income blacks and the working class.[53] The organization focused on nondiscrimination, issuing statements drawing attention to discriminatory behavior by local welfare offices. The national office was contacted by the Department of Health, Education, and Welfare to discuss ensuring equitable access to welfare benefits for all eligible recipients.[54] Although CORE was concerned with anti-poverty issues, it was not active concerning Kennedy's public welfare amendments.

As part of its new effort to include the poor in its constituency, the national office recommended various recruitment strategies to CORE chapters throughout the early 1960s. In preparation for CORE's national convention in 1963, Norman Hill, a field secretary, wrote to the Steering Committee recommending a Summer Project to be undertaken in the North.

> The purpose for a summer Northern task force project flows directly from the broadening and deepening of CORE's program—an attempt to develop a grassroots approach toward the elimination of the everyday reality of discrimination in the ghetto, an effort to involve people where they are militant.[55]

Table 3.4. CORE Prioritization of Anti-Poverty Policy 1960–1968

Organizational activities	Pre-EOA (1960–1963)	Immediate response to EOA (1964–1965)	Post-EOA (1966–1968)
Low-priority indicators (1 point each)			
• Position taken on issue (statement, convention resolution)		X	X
Mid-level priority indicators (2 points each)			
• Staff, or organizational committee, assigned to issue as one of several, or only, assignments			
• Internal evidence of funding for activities concerning issue			
• Communications to policy-makers about issue (testimonies before Congress or parties, position letters)	X	X	X
• Public speeches or statements by staff/leadership about issue		X	X
• National office directs local branches/affiliates to be active on issue		X	X
• Mailings to membership about issue			
High-level priority indicators (3 points each)			
• Fundraising with membership about issue			
• Mobilization of membership for actions about issue			X
• Consultation with policy-makers about issue (legislative drafting, implementation)			X
• National office offers workshops/training for local branches/affiliates on issue			X
• Internal discussions, as reflected in meeting minutes and transcripts, indicate issue as priority		X	X

Table 3.4. (Continued)

Organizational activities	Pre-EOA (1960–1963)	Immediate response to EOA (1964–1965)	Post-EOA (1966–1968)
• Organizational documents name the issue as a priority (resolutions, annual reports, org. publications)			X
• Organizational restructuring to address issue (overall restructuring, creation of new department)			X
• Organization offers own plan concerning issue			
No evidence of priority			
• Absence of any evidence of issue as priority			
*Priority level**	5%	27%	68%

*Priority level determined by organization activities as percentage of total possible activities. CORE activities during early 1960s totaled 2 of 37 possible activity points, a 5% priority score; War on Poverty period totaled 10 of 37 possible points, a 27% priority score; late 1960s totaled 25 of 37 possible points, a 68% priority score.

At the organization's 1963 convention, CORE delegates voted to consider socioeconomic issues in the future:

> [CORE resolves] to begin to think in terms of the future, giving attention the general area of our socio-economic problems and considering action on projects which would dramatize the root and extent of this problem.[56]

Although the organization did not embark on any national anti-poverty efforts as a result of this resolution, CORE's emphasis on socioeconomic issues and on expanding its constituency led to the organization's increasing attention to the poor during the mid-1960s.

CORE Attention to the EOA (1964–1965)

CORE's new emphasis on socioeconomic issues was evident throughout 1964, before the passage of the EOA. The organization testified at the Democratic and Republican National Platform Committees, and emphasized the plight of the poor in each statement. In his memo to CORE's National Action Committee outlining his presentation to each party, Norman Hill, program director, stated that he would include a list of demands on behalf of the poor in his testimonies, including a fair minimum wage, and collective bargaining for rent strikers.[57] In a public statement concerning the platforms of both parties, Hill singled out the Republican Party for its lack of attention to racial discrimination, and to poverty: "[CORE demands] that the Republican Party at its 1964 Convention declare itself for concrete measures that will solve the inequities of poverty and racial bias."[58]

The organization's statements before the parties indicate only a rhetorical commitment to advocacy on behalf of the poor. At CORE's 1964 convention, one month before the passage of the EOA, James Farmer pointed out that this rhetorical commitment had not been translated into the mobilization of low-income African Americans. Some staff and board members were concerned that CORE would focus too much attention upon poverty issues, and neglect the interests of middle class African Americans. Farmer, in his encouragement of the expansion of CORE's base to include the poor, attempted to assuage these fears by stating CORE's intentions to represent all African Americans:

> It should not be thought for one minute that CORE has no more interest in those who do not fit in the description of "grass roots" or "working class." There is no one Negro community . . . we want the involvement of every segment of the community which can be involved in this fight.[59]

After the passage of the EOA, the national office considered how it should respond to the Act, and if it should participate in its implementation. Staff were concerned that the poor would not be adequately involved with the War on Poverty programs, and would instead find themselves excluded from local program development. Because of such concerns, CORE had not yet arrived at a national position or strategy concerning the EOA by January 1965.[60] However, field staff and chapters had been actively overseeing the implementation of the program, and the creation of CAPs, since at least November 1964. The national office was aware of these activities, and felt it was important to at least send guidelines on EOA implementation to the chapters.[61] In February, the National Action Council declared that "CORE is deeply concerned about the status of public welfare in the United States and urges its chapters to engage in programs directed toward improving welfare services in their communities."[62] This statement indicated that the national office would support local activities, even if it was not pursuing anti-poverty campaigns at the national level.

Many chapters chose to primarily focus on anti-poverty activities during 1965. CORE officials were elected to anti-poverty boards in Newark, New Jersey, Milwaukee, Wisconsin, and Los Angeles, California.[63] In Los Angeles, a CORE field secretary opened a community office in Watts that offered job training and classes in African American history.[64] The Richmond, California, chapter hosted the "This Thing Called Poverty" conference in March 1965, and held workshops on mobilizing the poor and understanding the EOA. Additionally, local chapters organized protests based on the inadequate representation of the poor in San Francisco and Los Angeles, California, West Essex and Newark, New Jersey, Seattle, Washington, Baltimore, Maryland, and Buffalo, New York.[65] The chapters' role in the War on Poverty was often contradictory—CORE personnel would staff the CAPs, while at the same time voicing concern about the representation of the poor on CAP boards, and nondiscriminatory disbursement of anti-poverty funds. The chapters' focus on the anti-poverty program, and on ensuring the participation of the poor, reflected the local affiliates' overall shift of priority to advocacy on behalf of the poor. By 1965, most chapter offices were in low-income areas, and chapters primarily focused on community organizing activities (Meier and Rudwick 1973, 360).

While chapters continued to be active, the national office debated the organization's position, and role, in the War on Poverty throughout the spring of 1965. Although the national office issued explicit instructions to local chapters concerning their approach to the War on Poverty, national CORE never arrived at an official position on the issue.[66] Reflecting CORE's decentralized structure, chapters had the authority to act autonomously, regardless of the national position. Some national staff members were concerned that a focus on anti-poverty programs would take too much attention away from implementation of the Civil Rights Act, particularly if local CORE staff started to lead CAPs.[67] At a National Action Council meeting in April 1965, CORE voted that it must come up with a position on the anti-poverty program, keeping in mind the staff's reservations about the federally run program: "the government is discriminatory; there are complaints about the creation of another bureaucracy; . . . there is a bias against urban Negroes; . . . in most cases the program is tied within the existing power structure."[68]

These reservations shed light on the national office's hesitance to take an official position on the EOA, or to issue explicit directives to its chapters. While the anti-poverty program had the potential to benefit low-income African Americans, it could be implemented discriminatorily, and was a federal government program—any CORE group working on anti-poverty boards, or in cooperation with the government, would no longer be able to affect social change from outside the system. Despite these reservations on the part of some members of the national staff, CORE chapters were quite active concerning the EOA.

CORE's July 1965 national convention was titled "The Negro Ghetto—An Awakening Giant," and included workshops on community organizing and "problems of the northern ghetto."[69] Farmer's Report to the Convention reflected CORE's concern with the anti-poverty program and its implementation. He pointed out that the federal government would never be able to mount an effective war on poverty as long as it was spending so much on the Vietnam War, and that the anti-poverty program "has to be seen as no more than a tool, useful at times but inadequate at best to the job." The national office instructed chapters to be "constructive critics of the anti-poverty program . . . insisting that local anti-poverty boards be truly representative of the deprived communities and the minorities which they are supposed to help."[70]

In November 1965, in an unusual instance of explicit instructions coming from the national office, George Wiley, associate national director, informed chapters that the Johnson administration had announced its intent to begin to limit the number of the poor participating in anti-poverty programs. Wiley urged chapters to "send letters, telegrams, petitions . . . calling upon [Johnson] to publicly reiterate that it is the policy of the administration to continue to attempt to involve the poor in as many of the policy-making roles as possible in the poverty program."[71] In his press release on the president's proposals, Wiley highlighted the activities of CORE chapters in San Francisco, Philadelphia, Cleveland, and Boston, and indicated that those chapters would prevent any attempt to decrease the participation of the poor on the CAP boards.[72] Wiley's focus on the activities of chapters indicates that while the national office supported chapter activities, and sometimes sent directives, it was not pursuing its own national strategy. This lack of nationally driven activities is reflected in CORE's attention to anti-poverty activities—CORE continued to devote a low level of attention to anti-poverty activities during 1964 and 1965.

CORE's Shifting Position on the War on Poverty (1966–1968)

CORE's support of the War on Poverty had been guarded since the passage of the EOA. Between 1966 and 1968, that limited support dwindled further, and the national office's activities and statements against the federal government increased. During the late 1960s, CORE's overall ideology shifted from integrationism and nonviolence to one that emphasized the necessity of economic and political empowerment for African Americans without the aid of existing economic and political structures. In 1966, James Farmer resigned his position as national director, and Floyd McKissick was appointed in his place. McKissick ushered in an era of decisive action in relation to the anti-poverty programs.

Soon after his appointment as national director in March 1966, McKissick led rallies in Los Angeles, San Francisco, and Morristown, New Jersey, to protest "the inequities and ineffectiveness of the anti-poverty program" in those cities.[73] The *CORE-lator*, the organization's newsletter, announced that "CORE is becoming increasingly involved in the War on Poverty, seeking to implement federal anti-poverty programs in a way that will reach the hard-core poor."[74] CORE also advocated for increased funding of anti-poverty programs at the national level. In May 1966, McKissick charged that the OEO was retreating from its fight against poverty, and that the federal government was not funding CAPs adequately.[75] CORE participated in a national lobbying day in Washington to protest cuts in anti-poverty funding, and to advocate for a guaranteed annual income and job creation programs.[76]

McKissick sought to direct CORE in its shift from emphasizing "desegregation and integration to [emphasizing] complex socio-economic issues." The National Action Council, CORE's decision-making body, supported this shift, and the New Directions program was implemented in 1966.[77] The national office instructed CORE chapters to reach beyond their traditional constituencies: "we leave out most of the community and CORE chapters are often unrepresentative of the people they claim to represent."[78] McKissick called this shift Phase II of the civil rights revolution, and stated that national staff and local CORE leaders would be retrained to focus on advocacy on behalf of poor African Americans.[79]

Throughout 1967 and 1968, anti-poverty efforts remained a top priority for CORE. The organization was facing financial turmoil, as it had been since 1966, and activities were increasingly curtailed. By 1968, CORE's position on anti-poverty had shifted, and similar to SNCC, the organization explicitly rejected welfare, or any federal aid, as a means to lift African Americans out of poverty. Stressing the need for independence for African Americans, CORE introduced a new program that emphasized community development and the creation of new businesses within struggling communities.[80] By 1968, it was clear that OEO programs would only continue to be cut, and that the federal government had turned its back on its commitment to the involvement of the poor in such programs. To CORE, the drastic cuts to OEO funding demonstrated why the federal government should not be relied upon for financial aid to poor African Americans.

Between 1966 and 1968, CORE continued to prioritize anti-poverty issues and the mobilization of low-income African Americans. However, the organization faced increasing financial difficulties, and the number of chapters began to dwindle. Instead of relying on local chapters, as it had during the War on Poverty, the national office became increasingly active on anti-poverty issues. The national office's involvement with local anti-poverty boards, its press statements concerning welfare policy and

African American self-empowerment, and its activities at the national level, indicate that the organization considered poverty issues to be a high priority.

SCLC Attention to Anti-Poverty Policy During the 1960s

The SCLC did not prioritize anti-poverty activities until the late 1960s, when it organized the Poor People's Campaign. From its founding, SCLC focused on desegregation and voter registration campaigns in communities throughout the South. The organization was pivotal in the planning of the 1963 March on Washington, where King delivered his "I Have a Dream" speech. King's speech passionately and eloquently linked economic, political, and social freedoms for African Americans— connections that were also reflected in the SCLC's approach to social change. During the early 1960s, the national office was involved with state-level activities to deny rights to welfare recipients. As civil rights protests increased in their numbers and intensity in 1963, the SCLC conducted a fund-raising drive to support welfare recipients who were losing their benefits because of their civil rights protest activities.[81]

Generally, however, the SCLC was not involved with legislative battles until 1964, when the Washington Bureau was opened to advocate on behalf of the Civil Rights Act. Although the creation of the Washington Bureau increased the organization's participation in legislative activities overall, it did not increase SCLC's attention to anti-poverty legislation. During 1964 and 1965, the organization maintained a low level of commitment to anti-poverty policy—in fact, the SCLC's participation in anti-poverty activities declined from 16 percent during the early 1960s to 8 percent during 1964 and 1965 (see Table 3.5). During the late 1960s, on the other hand, anti-poverty issues became the SCLC's central focus. Arguing that economic justice should be the next phase in the struggle for civil rights, the SCLC devoted itself to the planning of the PPC in 1967 and 1968. The PPC would be a multi-racial anti-poverty movement pushing the federal government to implement policies of full employment, guaranteed income, and affordable housing. My measurements of priority changes reflect this shift. During the late 1960s, the SCLC devoted a high level of attention to anti-poverty issues, and participated in 84 percent of possible activities.

SCLC Attention to the War on Poverty (1964–1965)

After the passage of the EOA, the SCLC addressed poverty in its campaigns without making the issue a central focus for the organization. During 1965, it embarked on the Chicago Campaign, its first project in

Table 3.5. SCLC Prioritization of Anti-Poverty Policy, 1960–1968

Organizational activities	Pre-EOA (1960–1963)	Immediate response to EOA (1964–1965)	Post-EOA (1966–1968)
Low-priority indicators (1 point each)			
• Position taken on issue (statement, convention resolution)	X	X	X
Mid-level priority indicators (2 points each			
• Staff, or organizational committee, assigned to issue as one of several, or only, assignments			X
• Internal evidence of funding for activities concerning issue			X
• Communications to policy-makers about issue (testimonies before Congress or parties, position letters)			X
• Public speeches or statements by staff/ leadership about issue		X	X
• National office directs local branches/affiliates to be active on issue			X
• Mailings to membership about issue	X		X
High-level priority indicators (3 points each)			
• Fundraising with membership about issue	X		X
• Mobilization of membership for actions about issue			X
• Consultation with policy-makers about issue (legislative drafting, implementation)			X
• National office offers workshops/training for local branches/affiliates on issue			X
• Internal discussions, as reflected in meeting minutes and transcripts, indicate issue as priority			X

Table 3.5. (Continued)

Organizational activities	Pre-EOA (1960–1963)	Immediate response to EOA (1964–1965)	Post-EOA (1966–1968)
• Organizational documents name the issue as a priority (resolutions, annual reports, org. publications)			X
• Organizational restructuring to address issue (overall restructuring, creation of new department)			
• Organization offers own plan concerning issue			X
No evidence of priority			
• Absence of any evidence of issue as priority			
*Priority level**	16%	8%	84%

*Priority level determined by organization activities as percentage of total possible activities. SCLC activities during early 1960s totaled 7 of 37 possible points, a 16% priority score; War on Poverty period totaled 3 of 37 possible points, a 8% priority score; late 1960s totaled 31 of 37 possible points, an 84% priority score.

the North. While in Chicago to draw attention to de facto school segregation and public housing conditions, Martin Luther King Jr., its president, emphasized the importance of addressing the widespread poverty experienced by African Americans in the city: "But the schools are not the only problem that we must face. Thousands of Chicago's citizens are living just at the survival level. Nothing is more dangerous to a society than the existence of a large segment of the population who have no stake in that society."[82]

In addition to project-based work addressing poverty, the SCLC addressed legislative components of the War on Poverty. At the organization's 1965 Convention, delegates called for Congress to amend the EOA to provide for more enforceable nondiscrimination policies on the part of local agencies. The 1965 resolution marked the first time that SCLC had included specific policy recommendations concerning anti-poverty policy. However, because the national office did not engage in mobilization of its constituency concerning anti-poverty issues, as it had in 1963 to prevent protestors from losing their public assistance benefits, the organization's attention to anti-poverty policy was lower in the mid-1960s than it had been before the War on Poverty.

SCLC Prioritizes Anti-Poverty: The PPC (1966–1968)

In 1966, the SCLC national convention passed a resolution that called for the increased participation of the poor in War on Poverty programs:

> We call for the establishment of policies that would insure representation of fifty-one percent . . . of low income individuals on all local governing boards and executive committees [of EOA programs], believing that too long have too many programs to help the poor been controlled by people who think they know what to do for poor people better than the poor themselves.[83]

This resolution differed from the 1965 resolution in its emphasis on the participation of the poor. Responding to the Moynihan Report, the resolution went on to state that programs intended to change the behavior of the poor would not be effective:

> We appreciate fully the work of the main programs designed to raise the cultural and educational level of the poor, but these programs cannot be effective soon enough to deal with the problems that attend this society lest they be coupled with programs that will destroy economic paternalism and rupture the master-servant relationship wherever it exists.[84]

Although the SCLC passed resolutions concerning the War on Poverty in 1966, it was not active in its implementation. Resolutions passed at the annual conventions guided the organization's focus, but did not include specific action plans. The organization continued to prioritize its voter registration and desegregation projects—priorities not fully supported by all the SCLC staff. After a meeting at the Citizens' Crusade Against Poverty (CCAP) in January 1966, R. T. Blackwell, SCLC program director, wrote to King concerning the organization's priorities. Blackwell was quite moved by the meeting, and urged the SCLC to take the lead in the War on Poverty. Blackwell, who would leave the SCLC to work at CCAP during the next year, argued that the SCLC's money would be better spent fighting poverty, rather than continuing to work on voter registration activities:

> It [fighting poverty in the South] precludes SCLC from indulging in any project . . . that would require the spending of $40,000 to recruit 250 students or more than $500,000 to register less than 40,000 citizens. There is a much higher level of skill required of us, as well as a more economical use of our staff's time and abilities. I am convinced that the war on poverty cannot successfully be waged without the involvement of SCLC.[85]

The SCLC never prioritized implementation of the EOA, but devoted its resources to saving the War on Poverty programs during 1967 and 1968. On December 4, 1967, four months after the passage of the EOA amendments, the SCLC announced that it would lead a movement to address the needs of the poor to Washington—the PPC.[86] Bernard Lafayette, the organizer of the PPC, explained the basis for the Campaign:

> We began to take a look at the rural communities, particularly in the South . . . what's generally described as the Black Belt in Mississippi and Alabama, where there used to be large number of blacks working on the farms. More resources were spent on studying about them than relieving their situation. While Martin Luther King felt that he had raised these issues and talked about poverty conditions, he was getting a deaf ear. In most cases he would go to the location of these people in dire poverty in rural areas, the locations where they didn't have concern or political representation. The legislation and the policies that were put forth did not affect their condition.[87]

The legislative priority of the PPC was the repeal of the 1967 amendments to the Equal Opportunity Act. During the announcement of the Campaign, the SCLC stated that the national staff would be reorganized to focus on mobilizing the poor in ten cities and five rural areas to go to Washington to protest the economic and welfare policies of the federal government. The Campaign would include a month-long protest on the national mall, where a tent-city would be built and house hundreds of poor people (Chase 1998).

On March 17, 1968, the SCLC launched King's nationwide People to People tour to meet poor people, and to mobilize them to come to Washington. Over one month,

> Dr. King [met] with poor families in their rural shanties and slum tenements, walk[ed] the streets of America's ghettos, visit[ed] disadvantaged school-children, and [spoke] at mass rallies where poor people [presented] their grievances in hearings. The purpose [was] to . . . motivate people to join the Campaign for decent jobs and income and the right to a decent life.[88]

SCLC affiliates were responsible for organizing ministers, business leaders, students, and professionals to present donations at the mass meeting held during King's visit.[89] In addition to organizing for King's tour, the affiliates were primarily responsible for the fundraising and mobilization of the poor for the PPC.[90]

The organizational activities of the PPC were interrupted when King was assassinated in Memphis, Tennessee, on April 4, 1968. Because of his assassination, the Campaign's trip to Washington was postponed for a week, from April 22 to April 29. On April 20, the national office sent a letter to affiliates stating that "the Campaign should not be further delayed and we will continue [King's] work forthwith and make the Washington Campaign a great memorial to him." In the same memo, the SCLC announced the creation of the Committee of 100, two-thirds of whom would be drawn from the nation's poor, and one-third of whom would be national leaders. This Committee would meet in Washington on April 29 to begin meetings with various government officials.[91]

During the week of April 29, representatives from the PPC met with government officials from the Departments of Justice; Interior; Health, Education, and Welfare; Labor; Agriculture; and the OEO. Although tailored to each department's jurisdiction, the PPC's list of demands remained consistent: a food stamp program based on income, not family size; a guaranteed income; welfare reform to remove any work requirements and increase disbursements; federal funding for public housing renewal; and universal health insurance. During the second week of June, the PPC received responses from government agencies regarding its list of demands. All departments pledged to include the poor in the planning of anti-poverty programs.[92]

The second stage of the PPC was the establishment of a tent-city on the national mall. Resurrection City included a government, entertainment, restaurants, childcare, and classes taught by participants and organizers on topics such as nonviolent resistance. On June 19, SCLC held its day of mass demonstrations, Solidarity Day. Although only hundreds of people had been living in Resurrection City, 50,000 arrived for the protests on June 19. The mass demonstrations were the last stage of the PPC. At the end of June, police violence invaded Resurrection City, resulting in injuries to participants and numerous arrests, as well as damage to the tents and food.[93] The violence did not end, and one month later, on July 17, Ralph Abernathy, SCLC president, officially disbanded Resurrection City.[94]

Beginning in 1968, the SCLC wholly devoted itself to anti-poverty activities and mobilizing the poor. Economic justice had always been a concern for the organization, but was approached as a secondary priority to voter registration and desegregation. By 1968, anti-poverty was the organization's primary priority—it tracked legislation, mobilized the poor, organized a nationwide campaign and march, and attempted to work with political elites concerning the PPC's goals.

SNCC Commitment to Anti-Poverty Policy During the 1960s

From its inception, SNCC prioritized the mobilization of African Americans living in poverty throughout the rural South. Eventually, this commitment would extend to low-income African Americans living in northern cities. The War on Poverty, and passage of the Economic Opportunity Act, catalyzed SNCC to push for nondiscriminatory, and sometimes revolutionary, anti-poverty policy. SNCC's priorities reflected the organization's consistent commitment to economic autonomy for

African Americans. Organizational representatives moved into local southern communities to coordinate voter registration and desegregation campaigns and were consistently committed to local activism that addressed issues of poverty. However, SNCC's anti-poverty activities remained largely rhetorical until the mid-1960s. SNCC gave anti-poverty policy a low priority during the early 1960s; the organization participated in 22 percent of possible anti-poverty activities. In 1964 and 1965, SNCC participated in 41 percent of all possible anti-poverty activities. By the late 1960s, SNCC's level of activity declined to 19 percent (see Table 3.6).

SNCC Focus on Anti-Poverty During the Early 1960s

SNCC did not prioritize antipoverty issues before the War on Poverty, but the organization was concerned with economic issues. At the end of 1963, SNCC's executive committee met to discuss the organization's future. The Committee decided that socioeconomic issues should become the organization's top priority. SNCC was particularly concerned with urban areas of hard core poverty, and the Committee argued that if such poverty were to be addressed, it would have to be "systematically and not sporadically."[95] The staff decided that the organization's new focus required a rethinking of strategy—poverty prevents people from participating in direct action activities, organizers would therefore need to use new tactics to organize poor people. To implement this type of organizing, the executive committee decided that further staff education was necessary about the causes of poverty and its effects in terms of living conditions. By the end of 1963, SNCC was committed to increasing its organizational resources to mobilize the rural poor.[96] However, this commitment was reflected in plans for staff education, and remained largely rhetorical until after the passage of the EOA in 1964.

SNCC's Response to the War on Poverty

SNCC increased its advocacy on behalf of the poor after the passage of the EOA because it believed that the War on Poverty was a disingenuous attempt to address fundamental economic inequality in the United States. SNCC's interpretation of the EOA is not surprising, particularly because of the implementation problems of the Act, which often seemed to discriminate against poor blacks, and because SNCC had long been unexcited about federal poverty programs. Even before the organization analyzed the War on Poverty programs specifically, SNCC was highly skeptical that they could ever be effective in alleviating poverty.

Table 3.6. SNCC Prioritization of Anti-Poverty Policy, 1960–1968

Organizational activities	Pre-EOA (1960–1963)	Response to EOA (1964–1965)	Post-EOA (1966–1968)
Low-priority indicators (1 point each)			
• Position taken on issue (statement, convention resolution)	X	X	X
Mid-level priority indicators (2 points each)			
• Staff, or organizational committee, assigned to issue as one of several, or only, assignments	X	X	X
• Internal evidence of funding for activities concerning issue			
• Communications to policy-makers about issue (testimonies before Congress or parties, position letters)			
• Public speeches or statements by staff/ leadership about issue	X		
• National office directs local branches/affiliates to be active on issue			
Mailings to membership about issue			
High-level priority indicators (3 points each)			
• Fundraising with membership about issue			
• Mobilization of membership for actions about issue		X	X
• Consultation with policy-makers about issue (Legislative drafting, implementation)			
• National office offers workshops/training for local branches/affiliates on issue			
• Internal discussions, as reflected in meeting minutes and transcripts, indicate issue as priority	X	X	

Table 3.6. (Continued)

Organizational activities	Pre-EOA (1960–1963)	Response to EOA (1964–1965)	Post-EOA (1966–1968)
• Organizational documents name the issue as a priority (resolutions, annual reports, org. publications)		X	
• Organizational restructuring to address issue (overall restructuring, creation of new department)			
• Organization offers own plan concerning issue		X	
No evidence of priority			
• Absence of any evidence of issue as priority			
*Priority level**	22%	41%	9%

*Priority level determined by organization activities as percentage of total possible activities. SNCC activities during early 1960s totaled 8 of 37 possible activity points, a 22% priority score; War on Poverty period totaled 15 of 37 possible points, a 41% priority score; late 1960s totaled 7 of 37 possible points, a 19% priority score.

In the *New York Herald Tribune*, Chairman John Lewis stated: "Giveaway federal programs— . . . the inadequate War on Poverty . . . —all provide a mere Band-Aid for the gaping wound of economic injustice. The problems are so tremendous that individual civil rights organizations cannot handle them."[97] This recognition of the inequities inherent in the U.S. political system caused SNCC to focus on local relief and organizing because overhauling the economic system was repeatedly deemed to be an impractical goal by staff and Committee members.[98] Throughout its history, and culminating in 1965 with the creation of the Poor People's Corporation, SNCC preferred a strategy of providing poor blacks with the means to escape poverty, and argued that aid programs fostered dependence on the federal government, which could not be trusted to provide adequate benefits on a nondiscriminatory basis.

At the Waveland staff retreat in 1964, three months after the passage of the EOA, SNCC staff discussed how to react to the War on Poverty. Responding to an executive committee directive issued in September, a workshop was held on federal programs, with special emphasis on the poverty program; however, the staff at the workshop decided they did not have enough information, and that further research was needed before SNCC could establish its position on the War on Poverty.[99] The national office was asked to provide information about the poverty programs, and, as shown here later, began to devote resources to providing SNCC staff with up-to-date information about the ramifications of the poverty legislation.[100]

Perhaps most reflective of SNCC's critical view of the War on Poverty programs was its weekly publication, in 1965, of "Life with Lyndon." Responding to the staff's request for additional information concerning the federal poverty programs, Jack Minnis, a research staffer, wrote detailed analyses of the War on Poverty grants, and the players in the federal government who were responsible for implementation, or, "poverty warriors." In the "Life with Lyndon" series, it is clear that SNCC was highly critical of the programs because of the small percentage of funds that were being allocated to poor people.

> On January 17 Lyndon announced that $101 million of war-on-poverty money has been allocated. A total of $22,670, .02 percent of the allocations, actually went to poor people in the form of small business and farm loans. The balance, 99.98 percent went to poverty warriors themselves. A typical grant (no loans to the warriors—only the poor must repay) was the one to the Systems Development Corporation of Santa Monica, CA. . . . While Lyndon's head poverty-warrior, Sargent Shriver (he should know a lot about poverty—he was born to wealth and married even more) could only find $22,670 to put into the hands of poor people.[101]

"Life with Lyndon" provides a unique lens into SNCC's ideology concerning anti-poverty policy, and makes clear that the organization was unsupportive of the War on Poverty programs because of its commitment to improving the economic position of the poor, not because of a lack of interest.

The tone of the "Life with Lyndon" newsletters indicates the organization's attitude toward the OEO programs in general—one of disdain: "It takes the guts of a burglar to call a sewer like this the Great Society. But, whatever he's short of, Lyndon's always been long on guts."[102] Using stronger language, Minnis described SNCC's opinion of the Johnson administration: "And it's not that we don't trust Lyndon. We trust him. We trust him to screw the people every chance he gets, and to spend a good part of his time looking for chances. That's the Great Society in a nutshell."[103]

SNCC argued that the OEO should increase its disbursements to the poor instead of funding corporate projects. This theme was prevalent throughout the newsletters, and was consistent with SNCC's ideological commitment to providing the poor with the tools to lift themselves out of poverty: "if Lyndon had decided to give the poverty money to the poor, instead of to his rich and near-rich friends, there would be . . .

families who had a decent living in the US who hadn't had one before."[104] In December 1965, SNCC was forced to stop producing the newsletter because of the high costs of researching, printing, and distributing it to the staff.[105]

In addition to its newsletter, the national office organized protests against the slow implementation of War on Poverty programs at the national level. The Washington and national offices organized two days of protests in Washington to "break the poverty barrier," and demanded immediate implementation of War on Poverty programs. The organization indicated that the protests were "the first major unemployment demonstrations in the US in 10 years."[106] SNCC also focused on poverty alleviation through local outreach to help residents receive the appropriate amount of welfare benefits.[107]

Although the national office did coordinate a limited number of national-level activities, SNCC advocated that local organizations be at the forefront of the fight to gain improvements for poor people. In 1965, the national office prioritized a local anti-poverty project, the Poor People's Corporation. The Corporation's founding conference was held at Tougaloo College in Tougaloo, Mississippi, and included 300 participants. Jesse Morris, a SNCC field organizer, helped found the organization (Carson 1995, 172). Upon its founding, the Corporation identified the failings of the War on Poverty as one impetus for its creation:

> the poor are not being involved in the planning of the Community Action Programs . . . and . . . politicians are using the "War on Poverty" for patronage and other political purposes. In Mississippi, a new approach is being tried . . . A Poor People's Corporation has been formed. . . . This corporation is responsible for providing technical assistance to low income groups that have been formed for self-help purposes and to provide financial and other resources to said groups.[108]

The purpose of the Corporation was "to assist low income groups in their efforts to receive financial assistance to initiate and sustain self help projects of a cooperative nature that are designed to offset some of the effects of poverty."[109]

Reflecting SNCC's commitment to the distribution of anti-poverty funds to the poor themselves, the Corporation's entire budget was spent on anti-poverty projects. Every three months, members of the Corporation, who were residents of black communities in Mississippi, would review proposals and vote on the projects that should be supported by the Corporation (Carson 1995, 172). The funds of the Corporation were not to be spent to maintain the organization. The Corporation was staffed by one full-time worker, whose low wages were paid by SNCC, and three volunteers.[110] The focus on providing funds to the poor, and not on maintaining the organization, reflected the anti-bureaucratic ideology of many SNCC staff. Additionally, it prevented the Corporation from falling into the same spending trends as those of the War on Poverty, of which SNCC was extremely critical.

SNCC's response to the War on Poverty reflects both its rhetorical and action-based commitment to self-empowerment among African Americans. The organization did not engage with the federal government in its implementation of EOA programs, but rather served as a watch-dog to be sure that poor African Americans were receiving the benefits that were due to them. Additionally, the group helped organize local responses to poverty that would ideally allow the poor to develop a means for sustained income. SNCC's organizing activities at the local level are reflected in the mid level of priority it devoted to anti-poverty activities during 1964 and 1965.

SNCC Anti-Poverty Activities in the Late 1960s

SNCC's commitment to the alleviation of poverty through widespread social, economic, and political change was clear when the organization removed itself from the list of supportive organizations of the Freedom Budget. Written by A. Philip Randolph, the Freedom Budget called for full employment, a guaranteed income, the elimination of slum housing, government provision of adequate health care, and adequate transportation systems (Hamilton and Hamilton, 1992, 148). Although SNCC originally signed onto the proposal, which all national civil rights organizations supported, the central committee later decided to remove SNCC's support because "It is clear that there is nothing in the budget which deals with the fundamental institutions which cause poverty."[111] The Freedom Budget's approach to fighting poverty relied too heavily on the existing tax system, the same one that had created economic disparities in the United States:

> Our position is that the causes as set down by the Freedom Budget are merely symptomatic of more basic ills in society . . . It seems to us that people are poor because 2,000 families control 85 percent of the wealth in the country . . . In short, the Freedom Budget does not deal at all with the real problem—the fact that the economic and political institutions of the US have always either successfully resisted, or absorbed, previous such efforts to redistribute the wealth of the society. . . . We have to begin to ask ourselves why anyone purporting to sincerely propose a program dealing with poverty would suggest that the apparatus that created the poverty can be the moving force in eliminating it.[112]

In addition to such large-scale critiques of the economic system, SNCC maintained its commitment to organizing low-income African

Americans. In 1967, James Forman prepared an organizing brochure for SNCC staff, which focused on mobilizing poor African Americans:

> poor black people . . . have so much power, but that power is unorganized. It resides in you and me, but we must band together for strength. . . . We will tackle the problem of jobs, of income, of automation, bad housing, lack of quality education, welfare and the distribution of wealth . . . We must have organization at all levels.[113]

Later in 1967, chairman Stokely Carmichael reiterated SNCC's commitment to working with poor blacks in both the North and the South:

> we aim to bring the community a political awareness which does now exist on a mass basis and to the masses in the black community in this country . . . We are going to work with the black oppressed people of this country. They happen to be the sharecroppers in the South and the ghetto dwellers in the North.[114]

Although SNCC maintained its rhetorical commitment to the poor throughout the late 1960s as it faced organizational decline, its activities reflect the low priority given to poverty policy in the late 1960s. As SNCC faced increasing financial challenges, the organization could not maintain its focus on addressing poverty at the local level. SNCC's approach to poverty alleviation required substantial organizational resources, such as those devoted to the Poor People's Corporation. This finding does not contradict SNCC's statements of commitment to the poor—the organization continued to speak out concerning the needs of low-income African Americans, but was not organizing activities concerning anti-poverty policy.

Civil rights organizations varied in their attention to anti-poverty policy during the early and mid-1960s. While some organizations, such as the NAACP and NUL, advocated for nondiscriminatory implementation of the EOA and increased representation of the poor on CAP boards, others, such as SNCC and CORE, remained skeptical of the potential for federal government programs to alleviate poverty. The NAACP, NUL, and SNCC increased their advocacy on behalf of low-income African Americans in response to the War on Poverty. Although these civil rights organizations decreased their attention to the poor after the mid-1960s, both CORE and SCLC increased their anti-poverty activities during the late 1960s. Both organizations responded to threats to War on Poverty funding with heightened organizational activities to maintain, or increase, funding for EOA programs. The NAACP's and NUL's representation of the poor declined after the 1960s; by the 1970s, such advocacy was much less of a priority for both organizations than it had been throughout the 1960s. The different levels of attention given to anti-poverty policy by these organizations provide a unique opportunity to understand the factors that led to shifts in priority within each group. I return to this question in Chapter 5, after presenting my findings of priority shifts within the NAACP and NUL during the late 1960s and early 1970s in the next chapter.

Chapter 4

Civil Rights Organizations' Anti-Poverty Activities During the Late 1960s and Early 1970s

Figures recently compiled by the Office of Economic Opportunity show that approximately forty-eight per cent of the total program funds are spent for what is described as "programming for Black Americans." Assuming that these figures are accurate, it is fair to say that any unfriendly or disruptive action against OEO programs, either by the Administration or the Congress, inevitably will be characterized as action against minority groups.
   —Clarence Mitchell, Director of the NAACP Washington Bureau, 1971

Anti-poverty activism benefited from the civil rights movement and became integrated into the purposes of many groups during the mid-1960s. After the height of the movement, the landscape of organizations changed. By the late 1960s and early 1970s, newer groups were disintegrating and were not engaged in national level advocacy on behalf of the poor. The NAACP and NUL priorities were affected by these changes within the civil rights issue niche, and by the public and political backlash against the War on Poverty. In this chapter, I analyze NAACP and NUL activities after the War on Poverty between 1966 and 1968, and concerning the Family Assistance Plan (FAP) between 1969 and 1972. The NAACP and NUL both supported the legislation when it was first introduced in 1969, but opposed the Plan by 1971 because of its low benefit levels and work requirements (Hamilton and Hamilton, 1992, 179). The NAACP's level of attention to anti-poverty policy began to drop during the late 1960s; the NUL maintained its high level of attention until the early 1970s. Both organizations were active concerning the FAP, but neither prioritized welfare reform as they had during the mid-1960s.

As I discussed in the previous chapter, opponents to the War on Poverty began to gain legislative victories beginning in 1967 with the passage of the amendments to the EOA. Because of the alleged failures of the War on Poverty, President Richard M. Nixon proposed the FAP in 1969 as a new approach to public assistance policy. The Nixon administration argued that the state and locally run service programs implemented during the War on Poverty were clearly ineffective, and that people would be able to help themselves out of poverty if they were simply given cash (Berkowitz 1991, 126). Various forms of the FAP were debated between 1969 and 1972, when the provision finally stalled in the Senate Finance Committee.

The Nixon administration's guaranteed income plan was a response to perceived failures of the overly bureaucratic welfare system. Advocacy organizations, including taxpayer associations, children's rights organizations, various citizens groups, and the National Welfare Rights Organization (NWRO) pushed the administration to reform the welfare system.[1] Despite its guaranteed income provision, the plan never received strong support from advocacy organizations or either party. Welfare rights groups, such as the NWRO, pushed the administration to pursue a guaranteed income plan with a higher income and fewer work requirements.[2] Conservatives opposed the extension of benefits included in the Plan, and liberals worried that the federal benefits would be lower than existing welfare provisions in the states (Berkowitz 1991, 129).

My analysis of responses to the FAP is limited to those of the NAACP and NUL. By the 1970s, CORE's ability to mount any policy-based campaign, or to perform effective advocacy, had significantly declined. The organization maintained a small staff, had very limited financial resources, and only several local chapters (Meier and Rudwick, 1975 [1973], 425). CORE had shifted its ideological orientation to Black Nationalism, was working toward sovereignty for a black nation, and no longer supported federal government sponsored programs:

> CORE seeks to establish in practice the inalienable right of Black people to determine their own destiny; to decide for themselves what societal organization can operate in their best interests . . . CORE seeks the right of Black people to govern themselves, for themselves and by themselves in those are which are demographically and geographically defined as theirs . . . CORE seeks to bring into reality the concept of a BLACK NATION

WITHIN A NATION . . . CORE has been laying the groundwork for wrest-
ing control of institutions in Black areas from all whites.[3]

Although it did not experience CORE's ideological transformation,
the SCLC faced similar organizational decline during the late 1960s and
early 1970s. After the Poor People's Campaign, the organization faced
high levels of debt because of the cost of the Campaign itself, and
because of heavy fines levied during its Resurrection City demonstration. By the early 1970s, the organization had few affiliates, its national
office staff had dwindled substantially, and its Washington Bureau no
longer functioned. The organization was no longer mounting national-
level campaigns, and was not active on national legislation (Fairclough
1987, 394; Peake 1987, 297).

SNCC held its last staff meeting in June 1969. At this meeting, James
Forman resigned as executive secretary, and was replaced by H. Rap
Brown. The organization survived for several years after Forman's departure, but did not organize significant activities, had no phone, and no
full-time personnel (Carson 1995, 295). The FBI continued to monitor
SNCC's actions, and in 1971 reported that the organization had "not
staged or participated in any demonstration or disruptive activity, and it
is believed incapable [because of its] limited membership, lack of funds
and internal dissention."[4]

Because of the CORE, SCLC, and SNCC decline by the late 1960s, I
do not assess their activities concerning welfare reform during the
1970s. Shifts in national level attention to policy by any of the groups
might be explained by their overall lack of national activities. Although
both faced financial challenges, the NAACP and NUL fared substantially
better during this period. They maintained their local branches, and
were certainly engaged in national-level advocacy, including on behalf
of the poor.

The NAACP Response to Anti-Poverty Policy (1966–1972)

After the passage of the passage of the Civil, Voting, and Economic
Opportunity Acts, the NAACP focused its attention on issues of housing
discrimination, voting rights for eighteen-year-olds, oversight of school
desegregation, and passage of the Employment Opportunity Act of
1972, among other priorities.[5] As I discussed in the previous chapter,
the NAACP considered advocacy on behalf of the poor to be a priority
during the War on Poverty. Although the organization participated in
fewer anti-poverty activities during the late 1960s than it did at the
height of the War on Poverty, it maintained its mid-level of attention

during the late 1960s. By the early 1970s, and during the legislative debates on the FAP, the NAACP devoted a low level of attention to anti-poverty policy (Table 4.1).

NAACP Attempts to Save the War on Poverty (1966–1968)

As policymakers attacked the War on Poverty beginning in 1965, the NAACP advocated for the maintenance of anti-poverty programs. The organization also sought to increase its own participation in the programs, and expressed concern that it was not playing the role that it should in EOA implementation.[6] The NAACP considered the EOA to be an opportunity to reach beyond the organization's traditional constituency of the middle class.

> [The EOA is a] golden opportunity for the NAACP to serve the hundreds of thousands low income and no income people who exist on or beneath the level of poverty. . . . In our court battles . . . we advanced middle and upper income Negro families. Little if any benefits from these advances have filtered down to the teeming masses.[7]

Staff were unhappy with the NAACP's elite image, especially after the urban uprisings during the summers of 1965 and 1966, when advocacy in low-income communities was considered vital by civil rights organizations.[8] In 1966, the national office instructed its branches to coordinate a War on Poverty meeting to discuss successful implementation of OEO programs in their areas. The branches were to make "a thorough effort" to invite the poor—persons from families earning $3000 or less—to the meetings and to serve on branch committees concerning the War on Poverty.[9]

In addition to continuing its outreach to the poor, the NAACP maintained a close relationship with the OEO, although the organization remained frustrated with its lack of anti-poverty grants from the agency. Richard W. McClain, a member of the national staff, expressed his frustrations to Wilkins, and explained how and why the NAACP should receive "some of the millions of dollars being spent ineffectively in the anti-poverty program."[10] McClain provided technical suggestions as to how the organization could be administratively eligible to receive funds, and then went on to explain why the NAACP should be involved with local anti-poverty efforts:

> the NAACP [has] the ONLY READY MADE NATIONWIDE ORGANIZATIONAL STRUCTURE AND RESPONSIBLE PROGRAM AND LEADERSHIP, which if given the proper tools and funds, could very well mesh the gears of the entire anti-poverty program and give the direction and affirmative action of the grass roots level that would be meaningful and give the

Table 4.1. NAACP Prioritization of Anti-Poverty Policy, 1966–1972

Organizational activities	Post-EOA (1966–1968)	Family Assistance Plan (1969–1972)
Low-priority indicators (1 point each)		
• Position taken on issue (statement, convention resolution)		X
Mid-level priority indicators (2 points each)		
• Staff, or organizational committee, assigned to issue as one of several, or only, assignments	X	
• Internal evidence of funding for activities concerning issue		
• Communications to policy-makers about issue (testimonies before Congress or parties, position letters)		X
• Public speeches or statements by staff/ leadership about issue	X	X
• National office directs local branches/ affiliates to be active on issue		X
• Mailings to membership about issue	X	
High-level priority indicators (3 points each)		
• Fundraising with membership about issue		
• Mobilization of membership for actions about issue		
• Consultation with policy-makers about issue (legislative drafting, implementation)		
• National office offers workshops/training for local branches/affiliates on issue	X	
• Internal discussions indicate issue as priority		
• Organizational documents name the issue as a priority (resolutions, annual reports, org. publications)	X	
• Organizational restructuring to address issue (overall restructuring, creation of new department)	X	
• Organization offers own plan concerning issue		
No evidence of priority		
• Absence of any evidence of issue as priority		
*Priority level**	19%	38%

*Priority level determined by organization activities as percentage of total possible activities. NAACP activities in response to FAP totaled 7 of 37 possible points, a 19% priority score; late 1960s totaled 17 of 37 possible points, a 38% priority score.

whole program the breath of life that the government, industry and foundations have been searching and crying aloud for. After all, in essence, the anti-poverty program is literally a blue print of our own stated aims and purposes on a broader scale.[11]

In response to the NAACP's concern with increasing its receipt of OEO grants, Maurice Dawkins, Assistant Director for Civil Rights of the OEO, sent Wilkins a series of recommendations. Dawkins argued that many NAACP branches were unaware of how to establish their eligibility to receive funds, and that the national office needed to provide explicit guidelines.[12]

The NAACP's 59th Annual Convention in 1968 emphasized the importance of anti-poverty efforts. The delegates passed resolutions calling for branches to "be diligent in pressing local community action agencies for 'maximum feasible participation' of residents in all areas . . . and to be vigilant in resisting welfare paternalism and political manipulation of anti-poverty funds."[13] The NAACP also called on the federal government to make the needs of the poor its priority. A similar directive was sent to branches:

> It is evident that there is a dire lack of information regarding the intent of the poverty program; that there seems to be a lack of interest by members of the affluent society in this program and a seeming lack of involvement on the part of the poverty program staff, for the betterment of the conditions among the poor; . . . this convention direct[s] our branches and all other units of our Association to immediately conduct workshops within all poverty areas, for instruction and guidance in the total community.[14]

As it attempted to expand its attention beyond the interests of the middle and upper classes, the NAACP recognized its ability to influence the affluent to support the anti-poverty programs. The NAACP's work to increase its involvement with the anti-poverty program, and instructions to its branches to advocate on behalf of the poor, are reflected in my measurement of priority levels—the NAACP maintained its mid-level of commitment to anti-poverty policy during the late 1960s.

The NAACP Activities Concerning the Family Assistance Plan (1969–1972)

As is evident in Table 4.1, the NAACP's attention to anti-poverty policy dropped substantially between the late 1960s and the early 1970s. By the early 1970s, the NAACP was devoting a low level of attention to anti-poverty policy, and was involved with 19 percent of possible activities. The organization did monitor the FAP legislation, and testified before both houses of Congress, but its activities did not include mobilization of its branches or membership.

During the House and Senate consideration of the FAP, the Washington Bureau testified before committees and lobbied both members of both Houses. The NAACP was particularly concerned with the FAP's relegation of oversight of welfare provision to the states. In his testimony before the House Committee on Ways and Means in 1969, and again before the Senate in 1970, Clarence Mitchell, director of the Washington Bureau, highlighted the discrepancies in levels of welfare benefits among the states. He argued that any welfare reform proposal must include provisions for federal operation of the programs if the states did not meet minimum requirements:

> It has been our experience that many federal programs do not provide the intended benefits for those in need because of poor administration or deliberate intent to deprive citizens of benefits in some states. We strongly recommend that any plan of assistance provide for direct federal operation if a state is unwilling or unable to put it into effect.[15]

At the 1970 Convention, NAACP delegates passed a resolution on welfare reform, calling for a plan that would maintain a federally financed and administered system and create a minimum benefit level at the poverty line. The delegates also expressed the organization's distress with the state trend of cutting welfare benefits, and committed the NAACP to monitoring welfare cuts and their impact on low-income African Americans:

> We expressly call attention to those governors and welfare executives who have announced or instituted across the board percentage cuts to establish welfare grants which will ultimately result in hunger, sickness and death of poor persons. Therefore, be it resolved, that this convention and its branches and its proper associated staff pay particular attention to the serious publicity of the mistreatment of the poor which are black, and to lend the resources of the Association for corrective action.[16]

In the organization's 1971 annual report, the Washington Bureau reported that it was monitoring the FAP, which was in committee in the Senate.[17] The organization neither supported nor opposed the legislation, but rather argued that certain changes must be made before the bill was passed out of committee. Despite the NAACP's reservations, Wilkins was critical of African American members of the House who voted against the FAP:

> President Nixon, for the first time in history, placed his Administration behind a welfare bill containing a floor below which no family would be asked to live . . . I would be interested to hear [the Black Caucus members who voted against the FAP in the House] explain to Negro welfare families in the Carolinas, Florida, Georgia, Alabama, Mississippi, and Arkansas just

why . . . they . . . opposed a plan calling for a $2,400 federal floor under welfare payments.[18]

Eventually, the NAACP's insistence on increased benefits, mandated federal oversight, and opposition to work requirements led it to oppose the FAP as proposed by Nixon.[19] The 1971 and 1972 conventions passed resolutions emphasizing the importance of strengthening a federal welfare system and reasonable benefit levels:

> The NAACP reaffirms its position on Welfare Reform . . . urging benefit levels as follows: . . . elimination of categories and establishments of a unified federally administered and federally financed system based solely on need . . . minimum benefits for individuals and families beginning at the government-defined poverty level . . . federal supplements to assure that benefits are maintained at least up to present assistance levels.[20]

By 1972, after the FAP had failed to be passed out of the Senate Finance Committee, the NAACP was strongly critical of the Nixon administration's policies affecting low-income African Americans. At the organization's annual membership meeting in January 1973, Wilkins criticized Nixon's legislative actions. He

> charged the Nixon Administration with . . . condemning millions of low-income families to continued misery in the slums by imposing an 18-month moratorium on Federal assistance to meet their housing needs; curtailment, transfer or withdrawal of Federal funds for such Great Society programs as day care centers, legal aid for the poor, summer employment for ghetto youths, Community Action and Model Cities.[21]

The NAACP specifically criticized the Nixon administration's attacks on welfare programs, a strategy "which provided [Nixon] with a platform for pandering to the anti-black feelings of the white poor and blue collar workers by proclaiming to uphold the 'work ethnic' even while the cesspool of Watergate and related scandals spread . . . into the White House."[22]

Although the Washington Bureau was active concerning the FAP throughout the legislation's life, and the national office eventually criticized the Nixon administration, the NAACP's branches and membership were never mobilized. When an NAACP member wrote the national office asking if it had any materials it could send her concerning FAP, the office sent the request on to the Washington Bureau, stating that: the national "office has not published any material dealing with the Family Assistance Plan." Clarence Mitchell at the Washington Bureau indicated that his office had not published material on the plan, and sent the member analysis of the plan prepared by the Congressional Quarterly.[23] The national office did not focus on mobilizing membership, or branches, concerning welfare reform during this period, indicating that the organization devoted a low level of priority to the FAP.

The NUL Declining Attention to Anti-Poverty Policy (1966–1972)

As I discussed in the previous chapter, the NUL considered advocacy on behalf of the poor to be a top priority during the War on Poverty. Table 4.2 illustrates the organization's ongoing commitment to anti-poverty activities during the late 1960s. During this period, the NUL participated in 100 percent of all possible anti-poverty activities. By the early 1970s, and during the legislative debates on the FAP, NUL attention to anti-poverty policy had dropped to a mid-level at 56 percent. NUL gave higher priority to anti-poverty policy during this period than the NAACP, but the organization no longer considered it to be its central focus. Issues of poverty remained highly relevant—the organization was engaged with the development of urban policy, and urban development in urban areas with high concentrations of low-income African Americans (Dickerson 1998).

The NUL Struggle to Save the War on Poverty During the Late 1960s

At its national conference in August 1966, the NUL focused on its relationship with government agencies, the funding that it was receiving to implement War on Poverty programs, and on the needs of the poor that were not being met by the War on Poverty. The organization's Health and Welfare Committee named four "Pressing Health and Welfare Needs," and ranked concerns about the level of welfare payments number four: "[The NUL should seek] legislation to raise the level of public assistance grants at the state level to the recognized standard of living."[24] The conference passed a resolution stating the legal rights of welfare recipients and demanding that all those who were eligible receive their public assistance benefits.[25]

In December 1966, the national office launched a nationwide campaign to save the War on Poverty's Community Action Programs. If CAPs faced further cuts, the NUL argued, the poor would continue to "[get] the impression that in order to get anything, they have to participate in activities like rioting."[26] The national office designated January 1967 as "SAV-CAP month," an all-out effort by the national office and local Leagues to increase funding for CAPs: "The National Urban League is of the opinion that nothing can be more important right now than to help save the War on Poverty for which it labored so hard to give birth."[27] In June 1967 Whitney Young, executive director, testified

Table 4.2. NUL Prioritization of Anti-Poverty Policy, 1966–1972

Organizational activities	Post-EOA (1966–1968)	Family Assistance Plan (1969–1972)
Low-priority indicators (1 point each)		
• Position taken on issue (Statement, Convention Resolution)	X	X
Mid-level priority indicators (2 points each)		
• Staff, or organizational committee, assigned to issue as one of several, or only, assignments	X	X
• Internal evidence of funding for activities concerning issue	X	
• Communications to policy-makers about issue (testimonies before Congress or parties, position letters)	X	X
• Public speeches or statements by staff/ leadership about issue	X	X
• National office directs local branches/ affiliates to be active on issue	X	X
• Mailings to membership about issue*	N/A	N/A
High-level priority indicators (3 points each)		
• Fundraising with membership about issue**	X	
• Mobilization of membership for actions about issue*	N/A	N/A
• Consultation with policy-makers about issue (legislative drafting, implementation)	X	
• National office offers workshops/training for local branches/affiliates on issue	X	
• Internal discussions indicate issue as priority	X	X
• Organizational documents name the issue as a priority (resolutions, annual reports, org. publications)	X	X
• Organizational restructuring to address issue (overall restructuring, creation of new department)	X	
• Organization offers own plan concerning issue	X	X
No evidence of priority		
• Absence of any evidence of issue as priority		
*Priority level****	100%	56%

*NUL is not a mass-membership organization; these categories do not apply.
**Indicates fundraising in terms of receiving corporate or foundation grants.
***Priority level determined by organization activities as percentage of total possible activities. NUL activities during late 1960s totaled 32 of 32 possible points, a 100% priority score; in response to FAP totaled 18 of 32 possible points, a 56% priority score.

before the Senate Subcommittee on Employment, Manpower and Poverty that current public assistance to the poor was far too low, and that the War on Poverty was ineffective because its programs had not yet reached enough people.[28]

As attacks on the War on Poverty succeeded, and funding was substantially cut, the NUL reframed its organizational mission and priorities around the needs of the poor at the local level. The summer of 1968 marked the fourth summer in a row of significant urban uprisings in American cities. Not surprisingly, the Urban League viewed itself as having a particular obligation to respond to these demonstrations of distress.[29] In June 1968, the League declared a change in organizational direction—the New Thrust initiative:

> The burning and looting that have ravaged our cities are due in large measure to the unanswered cry from the people of the ghetto for a fair shake in becoming part of the larger American society. The Urban League must heed that cry with a renewed effort to turn its own resources, and indeed the resources and concern of all America, to that all-important task. This new thrust recognizes our contributions of the past while addressing itself to the challenges of the present and opportunities for larger service in the future.[30]

The national office stated that because it "must become . . . a visibly active force in the grassroots black community," it would undergo a significant restructuring to be able to implement such organizational changes. Under the new program, affiliates would apply to the national office for New Thrust grants to implement social service programming specifically designed for low-income African Americans.[31] At the NUL 1968 convention, Young emphasized the importance of fighting poverty, arguing that change could only be brought from inside low-income communities, and that the NUL would devote itself to helping communities achieve this change.[32] In 1970, Young approached the Nixon administration to provide federal funding for the local initiatives. Beginning in 1971, Federal Thrust initiatives were funded by numerous federal agencies and departments.

The New and Federal Thrust initiatives, while not singularly focused on anti-poverty policy, marked an important shift for NUL in its attention to anti-poverty policy. The organization's new attention to low-income African Americans meant that anti-poverty activities would be included in its priorities, without any particular re-thinking of goals and strategies. However, the new initiatives made local-level social service provision the NUL's main focus, a change that led to declining attention to national anti-poverty policy during the debates concerning the FAP.

The NUL Response to the Family Assistance Plan

The NUL devoted attention to the FAP, and was vocal concerning the Nixon administration's approach to anti-poverty policy. However, the organization's attention to anti-poverty policy declined between the late 1960s and early 1970s. As compared to its activities to preserve War on Poverty funding, the NUL devoted only a mid-level of attention to the FAP (see Table 4.2).

On President Nixon's inauguration day in 1969, the NUL sent him a 51-page memorandum concerning the urban-racial crisis. The organization recommended that the public welfare system be abolished and replaced with a guaranteed income plan—a plan the NUL had been calling for since 1966.[33] The NUL considered the welfare recommendation in its memo to Nixon to be particularly important because "national, state and local welfare programs [are] 'obsolete, punitive, ineffective, inefficient and bankrupt.'"[34] The organization specified that the proposed guaranteed income never fall below the poverty line, be federally administered, and

> [be] a welfare administration based solely on need . . . an inclusive program which disregards number in the family, age, or family composition; . . . a level of subsistence (based on family size and composition) that moves (in at least five years) to the poverty level, which would rise according to both changes in prices and the standard of living; . . . a system which does not force the poor to work or to take training merely because they are poor, but, in a separate program, gives everyone a chance at training for a job or a better job, and help in getting work. . . . [The welfare system should provide] enforcement, federalization, and adequate financial support for welfare programs already on the books, such as Medicaid . . . [and] stepped up effort to champion and enforce the welfare rights of those who need and are on welfare.[35]

The regional offices, in conjunction with the affiliates, were responsible for performing political activities supporting this position. At the 1969 planning conference, the national and local offices recommended that affiliates plan speaking engagements on TV and radio, community meetings about proposed welfare legislation, and newspaper interviews. Affiliates were asked to report back to the national office immediately after such activities, so that the regional and national offices could be informed about any necessary changes in strategy at the affiliate level.[36]

During his speech at an NWRO conference in August 1969, Whitney Young criticized Nixon's proposed welfare plan, but also asked delegates "to 'recognize what is good' in the President's 'inadequate' welfare proposal."[37] Throughout most of 1970, the NUL supported the FAP, but argued that its benefit cap was too low. Instead, the group continued to call for "an unencumbered income guarantee, federally financed and administered, as a solution to the nation's complex and controversial crisis in public welfare."[38] The NUL also opposed workfare, or any work requirements, tied to public assistance:

> It is folly, and dangerous folly . . . to perpetuate the myth that the poor must be forced to work . . . There is no need to codify inequities or make harsh, not to say, brutal assumptions about the poor. . . . Categorical distinctions must be eliminated and a uniform program established.[39]

Based on the recommendation of the NUL Health and Welfare Committee, the Board of Trustees decided it must finally arrive at a strong position on the FAP by 1971.[40] When Young testified before the Senate Committee on Finance, he spoke in opposition to the Plan. Recounting that the League had testified in support of the FAP in 1969, Young explained that "Since that time . . . the proposals have been constantly changing and many of the changes have detracted from the potential effectiveness of the legislation."[41] The League's opposition was based on the diminished financing of the Plan by the federal government, the level of the proposed income floor, and the Plan's work requirements.

In October 1970, the national office wrote to its regional directors, asking that they name one affiliate in their region to adopt welfare as its top priority, and to work in cooperation with the NWRO. The League's own preferences for anti-poverty policy were outlined in its Domestic Marshall Plan, which it re-introduced to its overall organizational priorities.[42] Based on the Plan, public assistance would become a residual program—unnecessary because most poverty would be eradicated. For the time being, however, the NUL argued that public assistance would be a critical component of federal government policy until programs, such as those outlined in the Domestic Marshall Plan, could be implemented.[43]

In October 1971, Jeweldean Jones Londa, the organization's Health and Welfare Secretary, wrote to Vernon Jordan, executive director, apprising him of the public assistance situation throughout the states. Londa wrote that repressive social welfare measures were being passed in numerous states, and that the League should be active concerning these proposals.[44] The NUL urged its local offices to respond to welfare crises, and also stressed the importance of national monitoring of state actions during this period of welfare retrenchment. The organization was aware that the political climate concerning welfare policy had shifted against support for public assistance policies. In September, regional directors had been

> [alerted] . . . to [the League's] renewed concern about current national developments in public assistance and requesting current information in regard to the situation in each region and state. [The League] . . . asked

for information on the relationships with local welfare rights organizations and legal services and the recommendations for League actions.[45]

One month after Nixon's 1972 State of the Union address, the NUL came out with strong language against the FAP, marking a change in the League's strategy. In his testimony before the Senate Finance Committee, Jordan referred to the "Family Destruction Plan," and harshly criticized the underlying assumptions of the legislation, explaining that they did not reflect reality for people living in poverty:

> The failures of this bill are rooted in the philosophy behind it: that poverty is caused by the moral flaws of the poor themselves. From this central assumption flow the major elements of the bill: that benefit levels should be kept at punitively low amounts; that recipients are not capable of managing their own lives and of making rational choices and so must submit to bureaucratic direction of their actions; that poor people do not want to work, and so must be forced to accept employment regardless of the nature and wages of such employment or of the personal family relationship that would be affected by employment.[46]

In a letter to the *New York Times*, deputy executive director Alexander Allen wrote: "The family welfare provisions of HR 1 [the FAP] are even more damaging . . . to the best interests of the poor people and black people than the present bankrupt welfare system they are designed to supplant."[47]

The NUL's executive committee recommended that the organization continue to speak out against the FAP because "a number of organizations will be looking to the League for leadership . . . it is important for the NUL to be very clear in its opposition to the legislation and why."[48] At the organization's 1972 conference, Jordan argued that the most important issues facing African Americans were economic, and that welfare reform was a critical economic issue:

> A major issue . . . is welfare reform, and here too, the actions of both parties and of the Administration and Congress have been weighed and found wanting. The gross deficiencies of the Administration's welfare proposals are readily apparent. But all hope of an equitable welfare reform bill has disappeared by the action of the Senate Finance Committee, which has shaped a proposal so destructive of human dignity, so punitive in its approach, so stingy in its benefit levels, and so racist in its work provisions, creating a permanent underclass of forced semi-slave labor, that it constitutes a blatant, vicious assault on the poor.[49]

Jordan suggested that all pending welfare proposals be scrapped, emergency federal relief be offered to the poor, and new proposals be drafted.[50] Despite the NUL's strong rhetoric against the FAP, the organization was not engaged with the activities of local Leagues concerning the Plan, as it had been during the War on Poverty. While the League was planning its New Thrust initiative during the late 1960s, the national office was highly engaged in anti-poverty activities. During the implementation of the New and Federal Thrusts, the national office turned its attention to coordination of the initiatives, and moved away from national-level advocacy on behalf of the poor.

During the late 1960s, advocates for the poor were consumed with attempts to maintain federal funding for the War on Poverty programs. The NAACP and NUL were both actively engaged with this battle to varying extents. The League devoted its organizational resources to saving the War on Poverty, while the NAACP focused on elite-level advocacy, but did not mobilize its local branches or members. When Nixon proposed the FAP in 1969, civil rights and advocacy groups were cautiously optimistic—optimistic because of their general support for a guaranteed income program; cautious because the proposal was coming from a Republican administration. As the proposal worked its way through Congress, organizations became increasingly opposed to the legislation because of its cuts in benefits. The NAACP made public statements against the Plan, but did not propose its own alternative. On the other hand, the League proposed legislation to implement a guaranteed income with benefits at the poverty line, and built support for this proposal through its opposition to the FAP. Despite their activities concerning the Plan, the early 1970s marked a decline in attention to anti-poverty policy for NUL and NAACP. For both organizations, anti-poverty policy became one of many priorities during this period, whereas the War on Poverty had been a central priority for both groups.

Chapter 5

Explaining Priority Shifts During the 1960s

[CORE] is of necessity in a transitional stage, moving from a small elite corps working in the interest of the Negro community and the broader community to a ghetto-oriented group seeking maximum involvement of ghetto folk in the drive to manifest economic and political power. If we do not make this transition effectively—if we do not navigate these treacherous waters successfully—the organization will cease to be relevant.

—Letter to James Farmer, CORE Executive Director, from James Peck, former *CORE-lator* editor, November 30, 1965

Throughout the civil rights movement, national and local activists gained deeper understandings of the extent and effects of poverty.[1] Activists saw firsthand the depressive effects of poverty on political participation—poverty interfered with the organizations' goals of voter registration. For some national organizations, like SNCC and CORE, this exposure at the local level pushed poverty onto their agendas. After the passage of the Civil Rights Act of 1964 and the Voting Rights Act of 1965, some civil rights organizers argued that economic equity should be the next step in the struggle for civil rights—the movement's recent victories would be meaningless because of the high levels of poverty faced by African Americans. However, not all activists shared this vision for the future of the movement. Some argued that civil rights organizations should focus on overseeing the implementation of the Civil and Voting Rights Acts, which would allow the groups to pursue similar goals to those during the early and mid-1960s.[2]

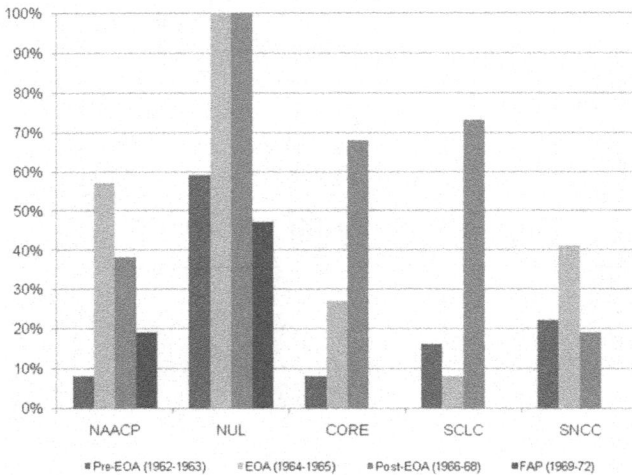

Figure 5.1. Organizational attention to anti-poverty policy.

On the other hand, giving priority to economic issues, and specifically anti-poverty policy, would affect low-income African Americans, and would indicate a shift in focus for the movement. Additionally, representation of the poor was an expensive endeavor during a period when civil rights organizations were struggling to maintain public support. Despite these disincentives, some organizations did devote a high level of attention to anti-poverty issues during the 1960s, and all groups at least considered whether they would give priority to alleviating poverty among African Americans. Figure 5.1 summarizes the findings presented in Chapters 3 and 4, and illustrates that levels of attention varied among organizations and legislative periods.

In this and the following chapter, I assess the factors that explain these shifts. Before discussing the factors that led organizations to shift their priorities, I present evidence concerning factors that did not lead to such shifts. In the next section, I consider whether changes in the groups' constituencies, or in anti-poverty policy itself, led the organizations to shift their priorities. Secondly, I analyze the internal and external factors that led the NAACP, NUL, SNCC, and CORE to increase their attention to anti-poverty policy leading up to, and immediately after, the passage of the Economic Opportunity Act. Finally, I assess why CORE and the SCLC made anti-poverty policy a priority during the late 1960s. My findings indicate that organizations' increased attention to anti-poverty policy during the 1960s was determined by interactions among internal structural factors and external factors such as inter-organizational relations. For example, the NAACP struggle to maintain relevance to the civil rights movement was precipitated by internal factors, such as the organization's historic elitist reputation, and the push of competition from other organizations for membership. These interactions led each organization to increase its policy advocacy on behalf of low-income African Americans.

Obvious Explanations? Changes in Constituencies and Policy

Perhaps civil rights organizations paid more attention to anti-poverty policy when African American poverty rates increased.[3] Based on existing literature, one might expect changes to an organization's constituency to affect its priorities (Clark and Wilson 1961; Moe 1980). However, as Figure 5.1 illustrates, each organization follows a unique trend in its attention to anti-poverty policy; therefore, as my findings in the next section indicate, shifts in levels of poverty and AFDC receipt do not consistently coincide with shifts in organizational attention to anti-poverty policy.

My examination of priority changes within organizations is based on shifts in their response to welfare legislation during four legislative periods. Another prediction based on existing literature might be that changes in the legislation itself explain shifts in organizational attention to the policies (March and Olsen 1989). For example, when welfare policy began to be devolved to the state and local levels, perhaps organizations decided to shift responsibility for the policy away from their national offices, to branch and local offices. In fact, my findings indicate that organizational attention to anti-poverty policy fluctuated independently from changes in welfare policy. I present these findings in the third section of this chapter, and argue that although funding was increasingly devolved from the federal level after the War on Poverty, national organizations had been involved with both national and local implementation of anti-poverty policy during the mid-1960s. Therefore, devolution does not explain steps away from national attention to welfare policy.

After presenting trends in poverty and AFDC receipt, and changes in welfare policy, as compared to organizational attention to anti-poverty policy, I explain how I assess the influence of internal and external factors on group priorities. In the second half of this chapter, I discuss the factors that explain shifts in organizational priorities. I find that internal structural factors, such as a national organization's relationship with the local level, will affect its perception of how to maintain its legitimacy in

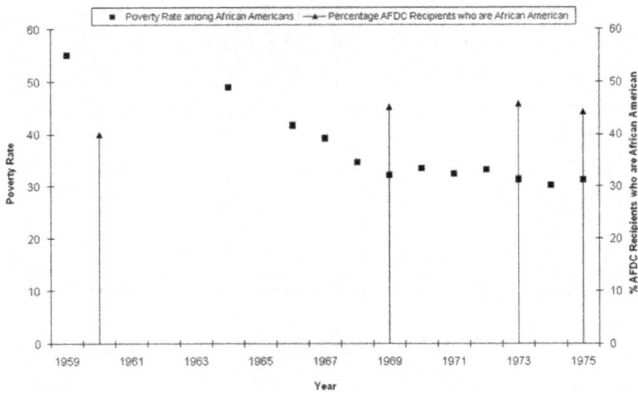

Figure 5.2. African American poverty rate and percentage of AFDC recipients.

the eyes of its membership or constituency. These internal factors interact with factors external to the organization, such as whether it is competing with other groups in its issue niche for membership, or working
to gain the support of political elites, to determine priorities.

Rates of Poverty and AFDC Receipt Among African Americans

Based on their mission or founding statements, the civil rights organizations I examine in this project claim to represent the interests of all
African Americans. Therefore, perhaps these groups chose to represent
the poor during periods when African Americans were facing rising poverty levels, or, specific to this project, were particularly affected by
changes in AFDC policy. In this section, I present the trends in the poverty rate and racial composition of AFDC recipients beginning in the
1960s.[4] Figure 5.2 illustrates the overall trends in poverty levels among
African Americans, and the percentage of AFDC recipients who are African American, between 1959 and 1975.

During the early and mid-1960s, the poverty rate among African
Americans declined as the level of AFDC receipt increased. Poverty rates
among African Americans had been dropping since the 1950s, largely
due to migration to northern cities, overall economic growth, inclusion
in public assistance policies, and increased job opportunities. Trends in
AFDC receipt during this period are tricky to interpret—the slight
increase in the percentage of African American recipients in the late
1960s was due to the increasingly nondiscriminatory distribution of benefits, not to increases in the number of eligible recipients (Lieberman

1998; Patterson 1994; Blank 1997).[5] Therefore, it is debatable whether increases in AFDC receipt among African Americans increased the relevance of the policy to civil rights organizations. The organizations would have also had an interest in the discriminatory public assistance system prior to the 1960s, even if the number of African American recipients was not increasing.

Between 1969 and 1973, the percentage of AFDC recipients who were African Americans increased by less than 1 percent, and the poverty rate among African Americans decreased by less than 1 percent. After 1973, the proportion of AFDC benefits going to African Americans fell, while the poverty rate among African Americans did not rise or fall dramatically. Based on these trends, often contradictory, it is difficult to predict levels of civil rights organization attention to anti-poverty policy. If the organizations' attention to welfare policy fluctuated according to the percentage of African Americans receiving benefits, I would expect the attention to consistently decrease during the 1960s and early 1970s. If trends in poverty rates among African Americans explain shifts in organizational priorities, I would expect attention to drop during the 1960s, and remain consistent beginning in the late 1960s.

Table 5.1 summarizes the trends in the percentage of African American AFDC recipients and poverty rates among African Americans, and compares them to trends in organizational attention to anti-poverty policy during each legislative period. As the table illustrates, neither factor explains shifts in organizational attention to anti-poverty policy. Poverty rates for African Americans were decreasing throughout the three legislative periods, and the percentage of African American AFDC recipients was increasing. Trends in organizational attention to anti-poverty do not mirror either measure of poverty among African Americans.

Between 1962 and 1965, all organizations except the SCLC increased their attention to welfare policy. Perhaps organizations, with the exception of the SCLC, increased their advocacy activities as more African Americans were receiving AFDC benefits. However, between 1965 and 1968, while African American AFDC receipt continued to increase, the NAACP and SNCC decreased their attention to anti-poverty policy, and the NUL level of attention did not change. Between 1968 and 1972, as African American AFDC receipt continued to increase, and poverty rates continued to decline, both the NAACP and NUL decreased their attention to anti-poverty policy. As this comparison between trends in poverty, African American AFDC receipt, and organizational priorities makes clear, civil rights organization shifts in attention to anti-poverty policy are not explained by economic changes among African Americans.

Table 5.1. African American Poverty Rate and Percentage of AFDC Recipients, and Organizational Attention to Anti-Poverty Policy

Period	Percentage of AFDC recipients who are African American	Trend in poverty rate	NAACP attention	NUL attention	CORE attention	SCLC attention	SNCC attention
1962–1965	No change	Decrease	Increase	Increase	Increase	Decrease	Increase
1965–1968	Increase	Decrease	Decrease	No change	Increase	Increase	Decrease
1968–1972	Increase	Decrease	Decrease	Decrease	N/A	N/A	N/A

Source: Trends in percentage of AFDC recipients who are African American and poverty rate based on rates in Figure 5.2. Civil rights organization trends based on author's findings as reported in Chapters 3 and 4.

The Influence of Policy Change on Organizational Priorities

Another possibility is that organizations adjusted their level of attention to welfare policy because of changes in the policy itself. In 1962, the federal government began to expand its role in welfare disbursements and service provisions. This expansion continued through 1964, and the passage of the EOA, which called for federal funding and direction of local anti-poverty programming. After the War on Poverty, the federal government began to decrease its involvement in welfare distribution, and to devolve responsibility from itself to state and local governments. Beginning with the 1967 Amendments to the Economic Opportunity Act, the federal government increasingly assigned responsibility for welfare disbursements, and funding, to the state and local levels (Weaver 2000; Jackson 1993; Heclo 1986). The Family Assistance Plan of the late 1960s and early 1970s reflected this shift—it lifted responsibility for social service provision from the federal government.

Based on March and Olsen's (1989) understanding of the importance of rules to institutional behavior, legislation, with the rules it imposes, may determine which issues an interest group chooses to prioritize.[6] Rules, such as the level of government primarily responsible for implementation of policy, may affect organizations' attention to the issue. Perhaps civil rights organizations determined their role in welfare reform battles based on the content of policy. When the federal government increased involvement during the mid-1960s, national offices were active on the legislation. As state and local governments became increasingly responsible for funding and implementation beginning in the late 1960s, national groups shifted responsibility for welfare reform issues to local affiliates and independent anti-poverty groups.

Although these arguments would support scholars' contentions of the importance of the rules and norms established by institutions, my findings indicate that changes in welfare policy alone do not explain the level of attention national civil rights organizations devoted to the issue. First, establishment of policy rules and implementation guidelines does not happen without opportunities for interest group involvement. Devolution of welfare programs to the state level has been, and continues to be, a contentious political issue. The process of cutting federal funding for programs that would benefit the poor is one that can be controversial and time-consuming and require the involvement of interest groups (Conlan 1998). It is unlikely that civil rights groups, which have demonstrated a historic concern with economic issues generally, simply declared the topic outside their realm of interest once devolution to states and localities began.[7] Second, the War on Poverty was a national initiative requiring local implementation. If national organizations were uninterested in local policy, they would have been uninterested in implementation of the War on Poverty, particularly because most were not receiving War on Poverty grants.[8]

Finally, civil rights groups varied in their level of attention to welfare policy throughout the 1960s and early 1970s. If devolution explains shifts in priority, I would expect organizations to devote their highest level of attention to welfare policy during the War on Poverty, and then to experience a steady decline in attention. However, only the NAACP and SNCC follow this predicted trend—the SCLC increased its activities as the War on Poverty was facing cuts; the NUL maintained its level of attention after the War on Poverty; and CORE continued to increase its attention to anti-poverty policy after the mid-1960s.[9]

Organizational Decisions to Prioritize Anti-Poverty Policy (1960–1965)

As the War on Poverty became a central priority of the Johnson administration, civil rights organizations responded to varying extents, and with varying strategies. As I established in Chapter 3, the NAACP, NUL, SNCC, and CORE increased their attention to anti-poverty policy between the early and mid-1960s. The NAACP embarked on a substantial, organization-wide priority shift. Although SNCC did increase its attention to anti-poverty activities during this period, it never supported the War on Poverty because it was suspicious of government programming intended to aid the poor. The CORE national office shared many of SNCC's concerns about the War on Poverty and support for federal anti-poverty programming; it was CORE's local offices that led the national office to take a position. As opposed to CORE and SNCC, the NUL consistently devoted a substantial level of attention to national anti-poverty policy—however, even the NUL surpassed its previous commitment to advocacy on behalf of the poor during the War on Poverty.

NAACP Protection of Its Preeminence Among
Civil Rights Organizations (1960–1965)

The NAACP's founding bylaws established the group as a highly centralized one whose activities would be implemented by its branches. Charles Flint Kellogg argues that "From the beginning, the Association was highly centralized and the national body maintained control over branches and membership" (Kellogg 1967, 119). The national office's authority to establish priorities does not indicate that there were no tensions between the national and local offices, or even that the local offices effectively responded to national priorities.[10] However, the national office unquestionably recognized its authority over its branches, and consistently worked to enforce its priorities with local offices. This internal dynamic stands in marked contrast to other organizations, such as SNCC, which struggled with whether the national office had authority to determine local priorities. For the NAACP, priority-setting at the national level applied to all organizational offices at the regional, state, and local levels.

As the civil rights movement picked up steam during the early 1960s, the NAACP increasingly worried about losing members to organizations, such as SNCC and CORE, as well as losing the public's perception of the NAACP as the preeminent civil rights organization. Throughout its history, the NAACP had come under fire for catering to the interests of the middle and upper classes.[11] This reputation led the organization to be particularly concerned with maintaining its relevance to the movement as poverty became an increasingly important issue for civil rights organizations. Gloster B. Current, director of branches, expressed NAACP fears about the actions of new civil rights groups in a letter to L. Pearl Mitchell, a Board member:

> Today there are competitive organizations in the field. . . . They feel that if they can carve out a role for themselves and thus diminish the strength and agility of the larger civil rights organizations in the field, that they will be able to corner the civil rights market and take control of it.[12]

The NAACP was quite concerned with the recruitment strategies of other civil rights groups. As the 1960s civil rights organizing intensified, and as the number of active civil rights organizations grew, the NAACP became increasingly concerned with its image as an elite, top-down organization. Newer, or newly radical, organizations were appealing to low-income African Americans, and emphasizing the importance of their involvement in the civil rights struggle. In 1962, executive secretary Roy Wilkins, reported to the Board that CORE, SCLC, and SNCC "all were in full-fledged competition with the NAACP throughout all phases of the civil rights program"[13]

Competition from newer civil rights organizations had direct implications for the NAACP's strategies. Before a staff meeting in 1960, which would address the NAACP's image, assistant secretary John Morsell received memos from national staff concerning the direction the NAACP should take in relation to political action and the masses. Mildred Bond, life membership secretary, wrote to Morsell complaining that historically, the leadership and membership of the NAACP had been middle class. Numerically, the organization continued to grow, but this was because the middle class itself had grown. Bond stated that the staff should consider whether it was time to break away from only middle class involvement.[14] Calvin D. Banks, field secretary, made a similar argument, and explicitly argued the importance of reaching a greater number of African Americans: "The talented tenth stigma must be erased. We must get closer to the masses. We must aim for a simplification of approaches which will increase awareness."[15] Herbert Hill, director of labor, agreed, arguing that the organization must focus on attracting membership at the local level to increase mass membership.[16]

In September 1964, after the Board voted to focus on the implementation of the EOA, Wilkins wrote a memo to the branches explaining the Board's decision. He instructed branches to immediately request representation on CAP boards to maintain the NAACP's visibility as the preeminent civil rights organization:

> As one of the Association's leaders, you will recognize at once that we are striking out in a new direction and launching a major new program area. You will also, I believe, welcome it as an absolutely necessary move if the Association is to maintain its leadership in our movement.[17]

Similarly, in its 1965 resolutions, the Board indicated that the reason for its prioritization of the EOA was to maintain the organization's leadership in the civil rights movement:

> NAACP branches can and should play an important role in mobilizing the Negro community in determining its representation in such local agencies [the Community Action Programs]. NAACP branches should be recognized as a primary source of those who represent the Negro community.[18]

The NAACP's directives to branches were driven by the organization's need to maintain its viability as a civil rights organization among all African Americans. In addition to its concerns about maintaining its reputation as the preeminent civil rights group, the NAACP was concerned with its own financial health during the early and mid-1960s. As Figure 5.3 illustrates, the organization's income declined between 1961 and 1962, and again between 1963 and 1964. This decline between 1963 and 1964 is not surprising—1963 was the year of highest contributions to all civil rights organizations, and all groups faced a decline in income after that year. The organization's membership also experienced a substantial decline between 1963 and 1964. Unlike its income trends, however, the NAACP did not recover its membership to a level greater that its 1963 level. Although the organization did not face life-threatening decline, the national office did have reasons to be concerned as income and membership levels fell in the early and mid-1960s. Because African Americans continued to face disproportionate levels of poverty, and other civil rights organizations continued to draw these disparities to light, the NAACP knew that it could not close its eyes to the needs of

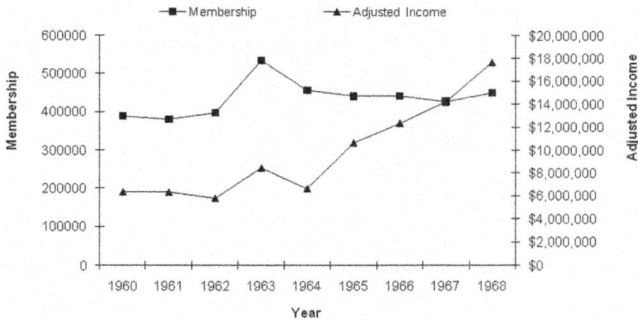

Figure 5.3. NAACP adjusted income and membership, 1960–1968. Income adjusted to U.S. dollars.

poor African Americans if it strove to maintain its preeminence within its issue niche.

The NUL Shift to Anti-Poverty Activities

Although the NAACP increased its attention to anti-poverty policy after the passage of the EOA, the organization did not receive War on Poverty funds from the Office of Economic Opportunity, and only began to strategize about how to receive such funding during the late 1960s.[19] In 1965, the NAACP Board decided that the organization should not become a prime contractor of the federal anti-poverty funding because

> tie-up with federal funds might inhibit the independent and critical role of the NAACP in protecting the rights of Negroes . . . [;] additional staff would be required for which there are no immediate funds . . . [;] there is some factual basis for concluding that there are political limitations on the freedom of control which can be exercised in administering the programs.[20]

The NUL, on the other hand, shifted its attention to the War on Poverty once federal funds became available. This shift was quick and dramatic—the League was restructured to match the requirements for War on Poverty funding and League leadership considered the organization to be the primary provider of anti-poverty services. As I discuss in Chapter 3, the League played an important role in the drafting of the EOA, and received assurances from the Johnson administration that it would receive hefty OEO funding after the Act's passage.[21] The reason for the NUL shift is not mysterious—federal funding became available to implement anti-poverty programming that the organization had supported since its founding. It is instructive, however, to examine the factors that allowed the NUL to engage in an organization-wide shift in focus. The national office's new emphasis on maintaining programmatic cohesion with its affiliates, its restructuring to facilitate this goal, and its commitment to its unique role in the civil rights movement facilitated the NUL shift to anti-poverty activities.

The NUL's Unique Role Within the Movement

As opposed to the NAACP, the NUL was founded as a social service organization. Therefore, it existed to provide services to, not political advocacy on behalf of, African Americans. The group was diligent about protecting its tax-exempt status by refraining from explicit political activities. Nonetheless, the League considered social work a critical avenue to social change, and one of its purposes to spark activism in its clients:

> It is not enough for the social worker to teach the poor how to survive on a substandard budget. The social worker must plant the spark and seed of change and indignation in the mind of every citizen in want. The social worker who is not a catalyst is a failure, and the social worker who does not urge reform will not be a catalytic agent.[22]

The League's commitment to providing services to low-income African Americans was strengthened during the War on Poverty. Because of its experience with social welfare programming, it considered itself unique among civil rights groups because it was "the one agency that has the know how to help communities draw up the kind of action plans that will change patterns [of poverty]."[23] The organization situated its commitment to education and training in relation to other organizations' approaches to social change:

> The Urban League is able to be effective in many situations which cannot be dealt with by other organizations. . . . At the same time, it must be recognized that certain stubborn problem situations historically have not responded to Urban League methodology. Some of these, however, have been successfully dealt with by litigation, boycotts, sit-ins, picketing, etc.[24]

As the civil rights movement gained legislative victories, the League moved beyond assessing its strategy as one that complemented the activities of other civil rights organizations. M. T. Puryear, NUL deputy director, indicated that the organization's approach would be the future for civil rights organizations: "I see a new role and direction for civil rights groups. . . . Picketing and protesting against injustices will go on, but many will follow the Urban League's lead in providing training to qualify the enterprising men and women who will march through the newly

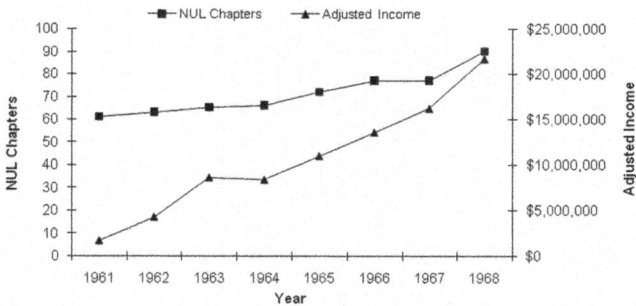

Figure 5.4. NUL adjusted income and chapters, 1961–1968.

opened doors.''[25] Puryear argued that civil rights leaders have an obligation to African Americans to follow through on legislative victories with such training. The destruction of racial barriers would be meaningless without providing African Americans the skills to take advantage of new opportunities, particularly in employment. Because of its social service orientation, the NUL argued it was in a unique position to offer skills training.[26]

The NUL's Strengthened National Structure

The NUL was able to translate its national-level commitment to the War on Poverty to an organization-wide priority because of the directive relationship between the national and local levels. When Whitney Young became executive director of the NUL in 1961, he sought to expand the organization, and to tighten the relationship between the national office and branch offices. Young identified the problem of too much autonomy for the affiliates, and argued that the NUL should be seen as one cohesive organization—not separate, autonomous organizations. Upon taking office, Young outlined how the relationship between the national and local offices would change:

> Both planning and implementation would be cooperative . . . National projects would be planned with locals and would involve them. Special projects that were discussed would receive final planning and implementation decisions would be made at a national conference, thus committing the various affiliates to work toward the success of the project for which they were going to be held responsible. (Parris and Brooks 1971, 399)

As Figure 5.4 illustrates, the NUL grew steadily during the early and mid-1960s. The organization's affiliates grew from 61 in 1961 to 77 in

1966; the NUL income also grew sharply during the first years of Young's administration. As the organization continued to grow, national leaders remained dissatisfied with their communications with local offices. The national office underwent a significant reorganization beginning in 1963—the Board voted to establish three regional offices in addition to the two existing offices:

> while the National office has grown in stature and the Executive Director has been accepted as a national leader, it must be recognized that there is great variance in the extent to which local Leagues are carrying our their responsibilities. Consequently, this new regional set-up is proposed to bring them closer to the national and to provide more direct supervision.[27]

This reorganization plan allowed for increased supervision of affiliates, alleviating the national office's concern that the organization's growth was providing the local offices with too much autonomy.[28] The Board pledged to hold affiliates to common standards of staff performance, Board participation, and programming. Affiliates that did not meet the new standards would be dropped from affiliation with the NUL.[29]

In addition to increasing the national office's oversight of local affiliates, the NUL specifically stated that its restructuring would allow the organization to "combat poverty and despair" through the establishment of a special anti-poverty unit.[30] Because of the League's regionalization, the national office was prepared to devote attention to the affiliates' activities concerning EOA implementation.[31] The regional directors were responsible for securing the League's participation in War on Poverty programming, and for ensuring that the League was represented on CAP Boards.[32]

Throughout the 1960s, the national office continued to strengthen the mechanisms to oversee the activities of affiliates. The NUL considered the implementation of War on Poverty programs to be its responsibility within the civil rights movement. The organization restructured itself into a politically active, nationally directed social service agency. Because of its increased national oversight of local offices, the NUL was an easy choice when the federal government was distributing anti-poverty funds. The national office was able to advise local Leagues in their anti-poverty activities, and to keep a close eye on affiliate activities through the regional directors—such oversight would have been very difficult, if not impossible, before Young's tenure and the changes he brought.

The case studies of the NAACP and the NUL reveal the importance of the interaction between internal and external factors in organizational priority-setting. Competition from external organizations with similar missions affected the priorities of the NAACP. The organization's structure determined how it implemented its new priority of advocacy on behalf of the poor. The NUL case also partially supports my expectation that competition will influence priorities. The League increased its attention to anti-poverty policy to maintain, and strengthen, its position among civil rights organizations. The possibility of governmental funding contributed to the League's decision to restructure to facilitate its implementation of the EOA.

Factors Contributing to SNCC Attention to Anti-Poverty Policy

SNCC was founded in April 1960 to coordinate the growing student movement throughout the South. Because other civil rights groups had to work to build local chapters and to maintain themselves as organizations, SNCC staff argued that these groups were not able to take risks concerning their programs and priorities. SNCC, on the other hand, conceived of itself as a coordinating agency that did not function as a traditional interest group, and therefore did not determine its priorities based on a concern with maintaining itself. SNCC did not build chapters at the local level; therefore, it could work to form "community movements" as opposed to "community organizations."[33] Because SNCC was committed to developing community and political organizations at the local level, it was particularly concerned with the implications of the high levels of poverty among African Americans, especially in the South.

Despite its founding commitment to decentralization, SNCC developed a national structure by the mid-1960s, which included communications and research departments. Such structural changes, as well as organizational growth, made some national staff concerned that SNCC had stepped away from its commitment to local organizing and had become an organization concerned with its own maintenance and growth. As Figure 5.5 illustrates, SNCC staff and income increased dramatically during the early 1960s. At the December 1963 executive committee meeting, staff discussed who its constituency had become. Although it was supposed to be southern college students, staff argued that "it is closer to the truth to say that the constituency is now the staff itself."[34] Despite such concerns, the national office continued to increase its oversight, and direction, of local activities throughout 1964 and 1965. Through firings of field staff, and increasing national directives about local programming, the organization came under tighter control by the national office in 1965.

Although the national office increased its oversight of local activities, SNCC remained programmatically committed to local organizing. Staff considered SNCC's commitment to local protest strategy to be one of its unique characteristics, as compared to other civil rights orga-

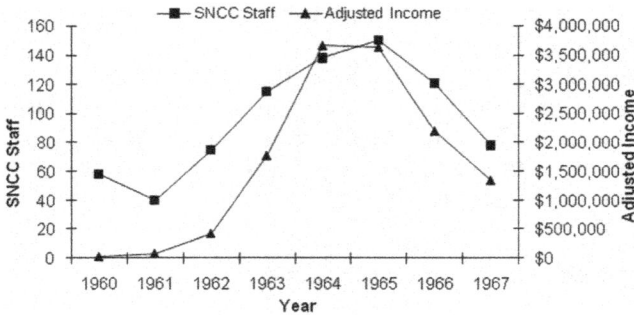

Figure 5.5. SNCC adjusted income and staff. Income adjusted to 2002 dollars.

nizations that were focusing on more traditional forms of political activity.[35] The group's focus on the local level, and local level protest strategies, was reflected in its organizing attempts. Through community building and mobilizing at the local level, SNCC argued that the black masses would be able to gain political control. While activities at the national level were sometimes relevant, it was local-level organizing that would produce the leaders necessary to effect social change: "In order for the Negro to keep his political power, assuming he will have it and assuming he will get the vote, there must be grassroots political organization through housing projects, neighborhoods, housewife organizations, the churches, the social clubs, etc."[36] It was only through intensive community-based organizing that SNCC believed civil rights advances would be able to reach the Deep South.[37]

SNCC's Relationship with Other Civil Rights Organizations

SNCC was aware of the importance of distinguishing itself from other civil rights organizations, and that its position within the civil rights issue niche needed to be well-defined. At a 1962 meeting of the heads of civil rights organizations in New York, SNCC was forced to defend its unique approach to local organizing to other civil rights organizations. Roy Wilkins of the NAACP stated that he believed that other organizations, namely SNCC, were attempting to push the NAACP out of the civil rights struggle. SNCC also came under attack from NUL executive secretary Whitney Young, based on its lack of traditional organization. Young suggested that SNCC and CORE merge, since SNCC did not serve a unique purpose. SNCC staff responded that the organization's commitment to local autonomy made it distinctive among other civil rights groups: it was able to "establish clear identity with the local community by living in it to the point where [staff] is no longer outsiders. It is only this way that we will be able to crack the Deep South."[38]

In addition to its unique commitment to local organizing, SNCC defined its role in the movement based on its militancy. After the heads of organizations meeting discussed above, the coordinating committee defined its intent in terms of possible competition with other civil rights groups: "our intent is not to be on a competing basis with other groups, but to assist them where possible to fulfill their own objectives. This may mean stimulating them to direct action."[39] After experiencing ideological disagreements with other civil rights organizations during the planning of the March on Washington in 1963, SNCC was encouraged to maintain its involvement with other civil rights organizations after the March by Eleanor Holmes, field organizer, specifically for the purposes of radicalizing the other groups:

> as the most militant of the civil rights organizations, SNCC has an obligation to keep its point of view alive in the [organizing] Committee and to seek to move it in a more militant direction. . . . [the Committee] includes the far richer, far more influential, and far more conservative NAACP and Urban League . . . SNCC should not abandon its radicalizing role at this juncture.[40]

SNCC's oversight of the implementation of the War on Poverty was driven by its commitment to local activism and autonomy, and its awareness of its unique role within the civil rights movement. SNCC was critical of the War on Poverty, particularly because it did not provide enough autonomy for the poor. The group's commitment to local organizing and its consistent support for economic programs that did not rely on federal aid were unique among civil rights groups. SNCC was aware of the importance of defining its own goals and positions within the broader civil rights issue niche. Similar to the NAACP and NUL, SNCC's perception of its place within the civil rights movement made the War on Poverty a priority for the organization; and its structure, one of local decentralization, contributed to its critical response to the program.

CORE's Increasing Attention to Anti-Poverty Policy

Similar to the NAACP, NUL, and SNCC, CORE determined that it must shift its attention to advocacy on behalf of the poor during the mid-1960s. However, unlike the other organizations, these pressures came from within the organization itself. National CORE increased its attention to anti-poverty policy after months of chapter activity, but did not give the issue high priority at the national level because of its federated structure.

CORE's Organizational Philosophy

CORE's reliance on local chapters for programming and decision making was evident from the organization's founding. Because it was founded as a federation of local groups, CORE's structure included membership only to local chapters, not to the national organization. At the 1958 annual convention, the national office added a new category of membership to the organization's constitution that would permit individuals to join the national organization. Associate members were individuals who supported the national office financially; but, unlike members at the local level, the amended constitution explicitly stated that associate members did not have input into the organization's direction.[41] Because local organizing was an important component of CORE's founding mission, the national office recognized the need to maintain local autonomy. At the 1960 Convention, Executive Secretary James Robinson remarked:

> It is . . . most important that the national convention as such not predetermine a large number of national action projects. Such predetermination would preclude flexibility: the national office would be so oriented as not to be of very much help in forming more locals, or helping existing local groups meet unforeseen emergencies . . . CORE is set-up to continue and expand local actions.[42]

As the civil rights movement gained momentum, CORE's structure was often frustrating to the national office, which attempted to centralize the organization throughout the 1960s. However, because of the established autonomy of CORE affiliates, the national office was not successful at its attempts to control local programming. In December 1960, the National Action Committee (NAC), one of CORE's decision-making bodies, which was dominated by national office staff, attempted to centralize the decision-making structure by creating the position of national director. The national office's attempts at centralization of power were met with opposition from local branches. In 1961, New York CORE presented a pamphlet to the national convention titled "The Control of National CORE":

> The crucial question that must come before the 1961 Convention is what steps should be taken to insure democracy within National CORE. . . . The delegates to this Convention MUST re-establish control of the National Organization by its active members through its affiliated locals. It MUST devise a Constitution that will prevent control in the future by any small group.[43]

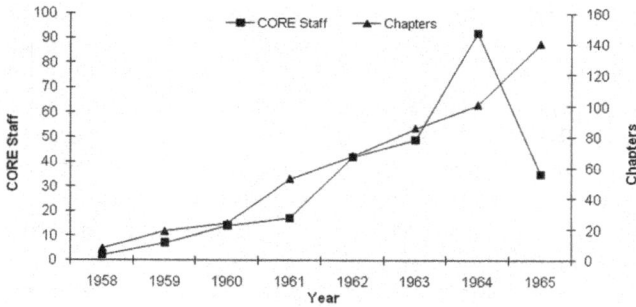

Figure 5.6. CORE staff and chapters, 1958–1965.

Because of such conflicts between the chapters and the national staff, CORE's 1962 reorganization further increased the role of chapters in decision-making—the representation of staff on the organization's decision-making bodies declined, and that of chapters increased.

CORE's chapter growth after the Freedom Ride in 1961, as illustrated in Figure 5.6, solidified the importance of moving beyond the organization's elite image, which the national office had been battling since the organization's founding: "As the branches have grown and extended, our roots have dug deeper too . . . [we] must broaden our base in the community, reaching the masses."[44] Because of ongoing rapid organizational growth, CORE's national field secretaries were asked to spend at least two weeks with new chapters to prevent organizational difficulties in the future, and to ensure that new chapters were able to attract the best local leadership.[45] The national office's concerns with its chapters increased as the organization continued to grow:

> The national staff is also aware of its responsibility as our chapters become numerous and more and more people join our ranks of active members. We feel a greater obligation to better service our chapters, to aid in developing clear project objectives, to provide more training in nonviolent tactics and CORE philosophy, to facilitate an understanding of meaningful civil rights program and to develop strong groups by advising local chapter leadership and membership in organizational techniques.[46]

CORE's growth led the national office to attempt to increase its oversight of chapter activities and programming. In 1964, the steering committee of the NAC passed a directive stating that local affiliates may choose not to participate in national projects presented by the national office, but that if an affiliate agrees to participate, it must do so according to the national office's program of action: "in no case may a chapter publicly oppose such a project."[47] This amendment to CORE's bylaws illustrates the relationship between CORE's national office and local chapters—before 1964, CORE chapters were able to oppose programs implemented by the national office. Even during a period of increased oversight of chapters, CORE remained a loosely federated organization.

By 1965, CORE had experienced four years of rapid expansion and ongoing structural changes. The national office attempted to increase its oversight over chapters during the early 1960s as CORE continued to experience rapid growth. Because of the founding commitment to chapter autonomy, the national office did not succeed in controlling chapter programming. Local offices implemented their own programmatic priorities, as they did in response to the War on Poverty, despite national office attempts to increase control.

Chapter activities and growth did affect national programming, however. As CORE continued to grow, the national office considered its relationship with local chapters increasingly important. It responded to chapter activities by eventually issuing guidelines, even directives, concerning the War on Poverty. As chapters became increasingly active in community organization by the mid-1960s, the national office recognized the need to move beyond the organization's elite image, and reframe itself as an organization equipped to represent the interests of African Americans at all income levels. Because of CORE's increased involvement with community organizing, the group increased its advocacy on behalf of the poor.

Overall, the case studies of the NAACP, NUL, SNCC, and CORE demonstrate the importance of the interaction between internal and external factors in an organization's determination of its priorities—the groups' decisions to advocate on behalf of the poor cannot be explained by examining internal or external factors alone. The findings indicate that organizations established their priorities based on the activities of other groups within their issue niche and that each organization's structure contributed to how it responded to that competition. The NAACP's perception of competition within the niche, and concerns about being replaced as the preeminent civil rights organization, pushed the organization to shift its priorities. The NUL, on the other hand, never felt that its position among civil rights organizations was threatened, and considered itself unique because of its historic commitment to advocacy on behalf of low-income African Americans. Beginning with the initial drafting of the EOA, the NUL gave priority to anti-poverty because of its historic commitment to such activities and its unique position as a civil rights organization committed to action and advocacy on behalf of the poor. Because the League sought to receive War on Poverty funding, it restructured its national office and affiliate structure to support anti-poverty programming.

SNCC also had a consistent commitment to advocacy on behalf of the African American poor. SNCC's perception of its importance to the civil rights issue niche, and its suspicions of federal programming, pushed the organization to vociferously critique the EOA. Political elites influenced SNCC's activities concerning the EOA. However, unlike the NUL, SNCC was not seeking elite support, and considered this consistent with its mission to speak out against the EOA.

CORE held similar characteristics to both the NAACP and SNCC. The organization was committed to autonomy for its branches, but became increasingly concerned with the activities of the local groups. Despite the national office's reservations about becoming involved with the implementation of the EOA because of its concerns about discriminatory implementation, local CORE groups began participating in CAP boards immediately after the legislation's passage. Through their involvement with EOA implementation, local CORE groups were successfully fighting the organization's elitist reputation. Because of the national office's concern with CORE's position within the movement, and the organization's decentralized structure, the group increased its attention to anti-poverty policy during the mid-1960s. CORE adjusted its priorities because of internal competition from its autonomous branches.

During the legislative period of the War on Poverty, at the height of the civil rights movement of the 1960s, each organization's perception of its role within the issue niche contributed to its decision about whether to give priority to the anti-poverty programs. This period was undeniably unique for the civil rights groups, and the groups' effect on each other may have also been unique. Perhaps during other periods, when groups were not perceived as working toward the same goals by other organizations, policymakers, or the public, the activities of groups within the niche were less important to each group's individual priorities. In the next section, I present case studies of the increased CORE and the SCLC attention to anti-poverty policy during the late 1960s. The civil rights issue niche during this period was experiencing upheaval, and organizations became less concerned about their own positions within the niche. Because of dramatic changes within the civil rights movement between the mid- and late 1960s, my findings in the following section complicate the effect of issue niche dynamics on organizational priority-setting.

Explaining Organizational Advocacy on Behalf of the Poor (1966–1968)

During the War on Poverty, some civil rights organizations increased their advocacy on behalf of low-income African Americans. However, as

Figure 5.1 demonstrates, not all organizations chose to increase their advocacy during this period. The SCLC did not shift its attention to advocacy on behalf of the poor until the late 1960s, when War on Poverty programs were under attack. The SCLC devoted all its organizational resources to planning the Poor People's Campaign. Although the organization increased its anti-poverty activities between the early and mid 1960s, CORE did not devote substantial organizational resources to such activities until the late 1960s. CORE's increasing oversight of chapter activities, and the organization's concern with its elitist image, led the group to give top priority to working within low-income African American areas beginning in the mid-1960s. For the SCLC, it was the organization's internal re-structuring and increased contact with local organizers that allowed the implementation of the PPC in the late 1960s.

CORE's Decision to Advocate on Behalf of the Poor During the Late 1960s

As I presented in the previous section, CORE's national office reluctantly increased its attention to anti-poverty activities during the mid-1960s as some local CORE groups were actively working to implement the EOA. To maintain its relevance to its chapters, the national office supported their activities, despite its reservations about the War on Poverty. By the late 1960s, the national office had become increasingly dissatisfied with the activities of the chapters, and worked to implement a national-level shift in priorities to increase the organization's relevance to low- and middle-income African Americans. Floyd McKissick, who became CORE's national director in 1966, emphasized the need for the organization to reach beyond its traditional constituencies, and to focus on the needs of the poor: "[In our local activities] . . . we leave out most of the [African American] community and CORE chapters are often unrepresentative of the people they claim to represent."[48] After the passage of the Voting Rights Act in 1965, CORE faced a decline in membership, chapters, and chapter activities. To reinvigorate the organization, the national office attempted to be increasingly directive with its chapters, and to emphasize advocacy on behalf of low-income African Americans.[49]

To implement this new focus, CORE embarked on its New Directions program, which was an ideological departure from CORE's commitment to integrationism and nonviolence. The program involved socioeconomic and political empowerment for African Americans outside of existing institutions, and required a coordinated grassroots political strategy by CORE's national office and chapters. Therefore, the national office sought to increase its control over chapter programming. Because anti-poverty policy was being implemented at the local level in a discriminatory manner, and because CORE had a new focus on community political empowerment, the national office increased its attention to anti-poverty policy during this period.

CORE's Transformation to a Nationally Directed Political Organization

CORE's attempts to increase national control over its chapters were frustrating for the national office, particularly because of the organization's historical commitment to local control. Local CORE groups did not easily acquiesce their programming to the national office and continued to implement their own programs, often without national office input—in 1966, the director of organization complained that chapters rarely reported any type of activity to the national office.[50] The national office's frustrations with its chapters were not new; however, as opposed to during the early and mid-1960s, the national office no longer struggled with whether CORE's founding principles allowed the national office to determine organizational priorities. Because of the grassroots coordination required by the New Directions program, the national office increasingly issued explicit instructions to its chapters. In 1966, the national office's position and suggested strategies for local CORE groups concerning the War on Poverty were issued as "instructions." CORE chapters were told specific policies to pursue, and how to engage in oversight of federal government activities.[51] By 1967, the national office indicated that control over local groups, and procedures to establish it, must be the top administrative priority.[52]

As CORE increased its emphasis on community-level organizing, the national office announced a new focus on political tactics. The group's commitment to political organizing began in 1965, when the national office established a Political Action Department.

> Why political action? An organized community is the most effective pressure group that can be created at the local level; it can form a lobby for legislation, can break a corrupt political machine, [and] can improve community conditions through political pressure.[53]

The national office instructed CORE activists not to become embedded in the communities they were organizing. Rather, similar to SNCC's strategy, they were to organize the community, and then to get out.[54] The national office emphasized the importance of providing communities with the tools to initiate their own political activities, and not to become dependent on the organizing skills of CORE staff.

CORE's increased attention overseeing the implementation of anti-poverty programs occurred because the national office was increasingly concerned with reports of discriminatory implementation, and because the organization considered local-organizing to be critical to its new program of self-empowerment among African Americans. CORE's national office gave increasing priority to anti-poverty activities as one component of an ideological shift away from concerns of the middle class. However, the organization's overall shift away from an elite focus did not dictate an increase in attention to anti-poverty policy. The national office's emphasis on local outreach and organizing led national CORE to increase its advocacy on behalf of the poor.

Factors Leading to SCLC Attention to Anti-Poverty Policy

The SCLC included economic equity as one of its concerns in its founding mission. However, this concern did not lead to action on economic issues until the late 1960s, when the organization devoted the majority of its resources to the PPC. As discussed in Chapter 3, the SCLC devoted few organizational resources to anti-poverty activities before the late 1960s—the group was focused on desegregation and voter registration activities. The SCLC's new focus on anti-poverty, as well as its public statements against the Vietnam War, led members of the civil rights establishment, the media, and the public to criticize the organization's goals.[55] Critics argued that civil rights organizations should focus their attention on the enforcement of existing civil rights laws, instead of extending the struggle against racial oppression to include issues of economic justice.[56] Despite these criticisms, in 1966 the SCLC declared that it would fight poverty on a national scale.

After the legislative victories of the mid-1960s, and the Watts uprising during the summer of 1965, the SCLC began to focus more attention on the situation of African Americans outside of the South. Specifically, the organization launched a Chicago Campaign, originally intended to assess levels of school segregation throughout the city. Through its work in Chicago, the SCLC became increasingly aware that levels of poverty, even in Northern cities without the histories of segregation in the South, disproportionately harmed African Americans, and perpetuated segregation. As I discuss in Chapter 4, the organization's leaders became convinced that economic justice must be a priority if legal equality was to be attained for African Americans.[57]

The SCLC's decision to devote its resources to a widespread mobilization campaign was based on its ideological commitment to economic equity, and the organization's new exposure to the conditions facing poor blacks in the North. However, such a commitment only determined the organization's concern with anti-poverty issues; it did not determine the SCLC's decision to embark on a nationwide direct action campaign. From its inception, the SCLC considered outside strategies,

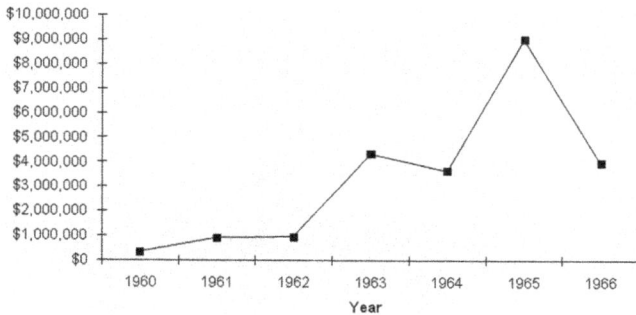

Figure 5.7. SCLC adjusted income, 1960–1966. Income adjusted to 2002 dollars.

like direct action, to be one of the methods that must be used in the struggle for civil rights (Garrow 1986, 85).[58] Each year at the SCLC's annual convention, the Board of Directors passed several resolutions advocating the use of direct action strategies. For example, in 1957 eleven resolutions were passed advocating nonviolent direct action as a strategy for numerous political goals.[59] The SCLC commitment to nonviolent direct action did not waver throughout its history, and eventually determined the method the group would use to mobilize the poor.

SCLC Organizational Expansion

The SCLC was able to launch a national anti-poverty campaign in response to cuts to War on Poverty funding because of its organizational and financial expansion during the early and mid-1960s. Between 1962 and 1965, the SCLC experienced substantial income growth, despite a drop in income between 1963 and 1964 (see Figure 5.7). The SCLC benefited financially from the public perception that it, and Dr. Martin Luther King, Jr., were central to the burgeoning movement during the mid-1960s (Garrow 1986, 264). The SCLC's increase in income allowed the national office to create the Department of Affiliates, the Washington Bureau, and Operation Breadbasket. These three departments would be critical to the development of the PPC, providing the structure for widespread mobilization and legislative activities.

In 1962, the SCLC launched Operation Breadbasket in Atlanta, Georgia—soon the program was operating in over forty cities. The mission of the program was "to find more and better jobs for America's Negro workers."[60] Operation Breadbasket institutionalized the SCLC economic concerns, and its Chicago office, directed by Jesse Jackson, was the organization's first nationally funded program in the North. Eventually, Operation Breadbasket's presence in the North was critical to the nationwide mobilization for the PPC.

In addition to Operation Breadbasket offices, the SCLC had its own local affiliates throughout the South. The SCLC's founding established it as a coordinator of local, community organizations:

> The SCLC is organized as a service agency to facilitate coordinated action of local protest groups and to assist in their sharing of resources and experiences. . . . The SCLC seeks to cooperate with all existing agencies attempting to bring full democracy to our great nation.[61]

Despite this mission, the national office established directive control over affiliates in 1963 with the creation of the Department of Affiliates. The creation of this department led to an increasingly coordinated relationship between the national and local offices, which would eventually be the basis for the PPC in 1967 and 1968; without a centrally directed structure, the national office would not have been able to attempt a national mobilization of local SCLC leadership.

The organization's expansion also included the creation of the Washington Bureau, which institutionalized its attention to national political issues. In February 1964, Walter Fauntroy, who had been the coordinator for SCLC activities in D.C. since 1961, became the Bureau's first director. The Bureau's opening indicated the organization's growing commitment to national legislative issues. Before this time, the group did not have a consistent presence in Washington, and was not particularly active on national congressional issues.[62]

By the end of 1964, the SCLC had achieved significant organizational expansion, and was ready to move out of the South, and to establish affiliates in the North. In 1965, the Board authorized SCLC expansion into the North in its annual resolutions, stating: "[The] SCLC will respond in an ever-increasing way to demands from Northern communities to provide assistance, and . . . a special study committee will be appointed to recommend structural changes necessary to accommodate this further expansion."[63] At a meeting of affiliates, the national office directed the existing local groups to assist in setting up local offices throughout the North, while the Department of Affiliates sent out mailings to active churches and businesses throughout the area.[64] The SCLC was able to establish an active affiliate in Chicago over a period of nine months because of Operation Breadbasket's presence in the city, and through Department of Affiliates contacts. Although the Chicago Campaign would be deemed a failure by the SCLC's staff and Board, as well as the press and the public, it did mark the organization's expansion north.

In 1965, the SCLC began to feel the public's waning interest in the civil rights movement financially. As I discuss in Chapter 4, by 1966 King and the SCLC were wrestling with the direction that the organization should take, in terms of finances, fundraising, organizational restructuring, and most importantly, program changes (Garrow 1986, 542). Bernard LaFayette, the SCLC staff organizer of the PPC, explains the organization's refocus on poverty:

> We began to take a look at the rural communities, particularly in the South . . . And we looked at the conditions that existed and all of the so-called economic progress we [had] made as a country. . . . These people [were] left behind . . . we looked at their plight and even though they migrated to have more opportunities, they weren't any better off. While Martin Luther King felt that he had raised these issues and talked about these conditions, he was getting a deaf ear . . . he would go to the location of these people in dire poverty in rural areas, the locations where they didn't have political representation. [T]he [civil and voting rights] legislation and the policies that were put forth did not affect their condition.[65]

By 1967, it was clear to the SCLC board and executive staff that organizational restructuring was necessary to maintain the group's vitality, and to implement the organization's new focus on poverty. King announced that a "sweeping reorganization" of the SCLC would include the "appointment of two new key executives, and the expansion of SCLC's field and administrative staff." Claiming increased need for professional leadership and technical skills, King explained that the expansion would allow for the organization of the PPC, the SCLC's newest priority.[66]

As the organization shifted its focus to the PPC, it was in a precarious financial, staff, and programmatic position. Until three months before the launching of the Campaign, the SCLC had been shrinking financially, and its programmatic focus continued to be debated by local and national staff. The expansion critical to the PPC occurred between 1962 and 1965; without the Department of Affiliates, Washington Bureau, and Operation Breadbasket, the national office would not have had the capacity to embark on such an extensive campaign.

Certainly, the SCLC staff's exposure to conditions of poverty among African Americans living in northern cities, as well as the organization's mounting concerns about the conditions contributing to the urban uprisings of the mid-1960s, pointed to the importance of addressing and alleviating poverty among African Americans. However, without particular internal conditions, this general organizational concern with poverty would not have translated into a nationwide direct action campaign. The SCLC expansion after 1962 insured that the organization had a national presence by 1968, providing the structure necessary to wage the PPC. The SCLC organizing tactics for the PPC indicate that the existence of a nationally directed affiliate network was critical to the movement's mobilization of the poor. Because of the development and growth of the organization prior to 1967, the mechanisms were in place to activate local leaders throughout the country to raise funds for the Campaign, and to reach out to the poor to attend the protest in Washington.

Conclusions

The case studies of organizational priority shifts to anti-poverty policy during the 1960s indicate the importance of both external and internal factors to decision-making. Specifically, the case studies point to the importance of organizational structures, and the relationship between national and local offices, to determining how and whether each organization would increase its attention to anti-poverty policy during the 1960s. The NAACP, which was very centralized, responded to the activities of SNCC, an external group working at the grassroots level. For CORE, the NUL, and the SCLC, groups that had maintained autonomous affiliates, this influence came from each organization's affiliates.

For each civil rights group, structural change interacted with external factors to determine priority shifts, indicating that organizations consider the activities of other groups within their issue niche as they determine their priorities. During the mid-1960s, each organization's position within the issue niche determined its response to the War on Poverty. However, as the civil rights issue niche experienced a period of upheaval during the late 1960s, neither CORE nor the SCLC were particularly concerned with other groups in their decisions to increase their attention to anti-poverty policy. Instead, both organizations increased their anti-poverty activities as part of organization-wide campaigns driven by changes in the political environments.

The NUL was influential in the drafting of the EOA, and maintained its influence with government officials throughout the War on Poverty. The League's relationship with political elites certainly influenced its priorities and its decision to commit itself to the War on Poverty. Additionally, the Johnson administration's declaration of the War on Poverty moved SNCC to staunchly oppose the federal programming, particularly because of its ongoing suspicion of federal government programming.

In the next chapter, I approach understanding organizational priority shifts from a different perspective. As I establish in Chapter 4, both the NAACP and NUL decreased their attention to national anti-poverty policy during the early 1970s. By the 1970s, the civil rights issue niche had re-settled after its upheaval during the late 1960s. The NAACP was secure in its position of preeminence within the niche. Once again, this position determined organizational attention to anti-poverty policy—this time, the NAACP's decreasing advocacy on behalf of the poor. Similar to during the War on Poverty, the NUL's implemented an organization-wide restructuring based on its receipt of federal funding. Despite its ongoing attention to poverty issues, the organization decreased its attention to national policy because of its rethinking of its strategies and purpose.

Chapter 6

Explaining Priority Shifts During the Early 1970s

A few years ago, the intensive and popular crusades of black activists forced the traditionally moderate NAACP grudgingly to become more militant. But now that the competition has been wiped out by death, defeat, prosecution, disappearance and exile, the moderates find it safe to resume their old posture.
—Clayton Fritchey, *Chicago Tribune*, July 18, 1971, A5

Beginning in the late 1960s, and certainly by the early 1970s, the universe of civil rights organizations had changed a great deal—SNCC held its last staff meeting in 1969, and CORE and SCLC were no longer mounting national-level campaigns. The NAACP and NUL fared better during this period, although both were facing financial challenges. Due to such challenges, changes in the civil rights issue niche, and political and economic changes, both NUL and NAACP decreased their attention to anti-poverty policy between the late 1960s and early 1970s.[1]

Consistent with my findings thus far, in this chapter I argue that external and internal factors interacted to lead both the NAACP and NUL to shift their priorities away from anti-poverty activities at the national level. For the NAACP, the decline of radical organizations allowed the group to feel secure in its preeminence within the civil rights issue niche. This security, coupled with declining organizational income, led the NAACP to revert to its more traditional strategies and priorities. The NAACP did not neglect social welfare policy overall, and continued to focus on litigation concerning employment discrimination (Hamilton and Hamilton, 1997). However, the organization was no longer focused on anti-poverty policy as a priority. The NUL, on the other hand, devoted itself to community-building within low-income African American areas during this period. It may seem counterintuitive that the NUL decreased its attention to anti-poverty policy at the same time that it was re-focusing its social service provision to low-income African Americans. In fact, because the national League became almost wholly focused on working with, and strengthening, local offices to provide social services to the poor, its attention to national level policy declined substantially. Because of the League's assessment of the political climate, and its concern with the urban uprisings of the mid- to late 1960s, the organization shifted its attention away from national-level policy advocacy on behalf of low-income African Americans.

Factors Contributing to Declining NAACP Advocacy on Behalf of the Poor (1969–1972)

In the preceding chapter, I presented my findings indicating that the NAACP strategically increased its attention to the poor during the War on Poverty because of the activities of other civil rights organizations. The NAACP perceived itself to be competing with these groups for constituencies, and for organizational preeminence within its issue niche. Because of the organization's nationally directed structure, the national office was able to instruct local affiliates to implement its new anti-poverty priorities without the interference of significant philosophical challenges to its leadership. As it did after the War on Poverty, the organization's attention to anti-poverty policy continued to decline between the late 1960s and early 1970s. By the early 1970s, the NAACP's attention to anti-poverty policy had dropped to 50 percent of what it had been during the late 1960s (see Table 6.1). As the number and strength of radical groups within the issue niche declined, the NAACP's preeminence among groups was unthreatened, and the organization was not tempted to shift its priorities because of the remaining radical groups. Its own financial difficulties during this period contributed to the organization's disinterest in expensive mass-organizing campaigns that required activities beyond its traditional strategies and priorities.

NAACP Relations with Other Civil Rights Groups

By the early 1970s, NAACP concerns about competition from other civil rights groups had calmed. The group's strength and longevity as compared to other groups was frequently reported in the national media. In a 1971 article about the future of civil rights leadership, the *Los Angeles*

Table 6.1. Decreases in Attention to Anti-Poverty Policy: All Organizations, All Legislative Periods

Period of change	Organization experiencing decrease in attention	Period 1 level of attention	Period 2 level of attention	% change	% change in attention
Period 1: early 1960s (1960–1963)	SCLC	16%	8%	−8%	−50%
Period 2: War on Poverty (1964–1966)					
Period 1: War on Poverty (1964–1966)	NAACP	57%	38%	−19%	−66%
Period 2: late 1960s (1966–1968)					
	SNCC	41%	19%	−22%	−46%
Period 1: late 1960s (1966–1968)	NAACP	38%	19%	−19%	−50%
Period 2: early 1970s (1969–1973)					
	NUL	100%	47%	−53%	−47%

Source: Levels of organizational attention to Anti-Poverty policy established in Chapters 2 and 3.

Times named the NAACP as the only organization whose leadership had remained intact:

> Of the old civil rights triumvirate of the 1960s, only the leadership of the NAACP—Roy Wilkins, Clarence Mitchell, Bishop S. G. Spottswood—has remained intact. Simultaneously no fewer than 40 national figures—from Malcolm X to Stokely Carmichael to Dr. Martin Luther King—have either died or been displaced or have declined in popularity.[2]

In January 1972, the *Chicago Tribune* reported that the NAACP was ranked as the premier, and most respected, civil rights organization in a Harris poll.[3] The organization had reason to be concerned about African Americans' changing perception of its importance during the 1960s. In 1963, 75 percent of African Americans surveyed indicated that the NAACP was doing an "excellent job" in "the fight for Negro rights."[4] By 1966, only 38 percent of African Americans indicated that the NAACP was doing an "excellent job."[5]

The NAACP's moderate reputation led to support from whites and the mainstream press, as concerns about Black Nationalism became increasingly entrenched during this period: "the NAACP now stands along among major national civil rights organizations as the symbol of the moderate, nonmilitant approach."[6] The organization distanced itself from Black Nationalist ideology, and explicitly rejected Black Power as a form of separatism, as Roy Wilkins explained:

> No matter how often it was clarified and clarified again, "black power" in the quick, uncritical, and highly emotional adoption it received from some segments of a beleaguered people could mean in the end only black death. I meant to have none of it. It was the raging of race against race solely on the basis of color. . . . What the NAACP wanted, what I wanted, was to include Negro Americans in the nation's life, not the exclude them. . . . The task of winning our share was not the easy one of disengagement and flight but the hard one of work, or short as well as long jumps, of disappointment—and of sweet success."[7]

The ideological commitment to Black Power by some civil rights groups caused the NAACP to reexamine its requirements for financial and programmatic cooperation with other organizations.[8] The 1970 NAACP Convention passed a resolution stating that any cooperative relationship should not compromise the NAACP's identity, and that "NAACP officials must differentiate between racism, separatism, and race pride. . . . We favor the fostering of race pride among the black people of America. We are opposed to projects and slogans which advocate racism, separatism and hate."[9]

The NAACP did not hesitate to publicly separate itself from organizations that did not meet its requirements for a cooperative relationship.

CORE, which had once been at the forefront of the integrationist tactics espoused by the NAACP, had shifted its ideology to one of Black Nationalism by 1969 and 1970. Roy Innis, executive director, publicly criticized the NAACP's tactics and purpose. In an article in the *Manhattan Tribune* on November 28, 1970, Innis wrote:

> It is well known among Blacks today that the NAACP is outmoded, outdated and an outrageous affront to the 30 million Blacks of this country. . . . The NAACP's chief reason for existence is to satisfy white needs and diffuse white guilt. It is not geared to meet the real goals of Black people.[10]

The NAACP responded with equally strong language: "Roy Innis' characteristic mishmash of half-baked philosophy, twisted logic and wearisome bombast is matched only by his ignorance or disregard of the facts."[11]

During the mid-1960s, such a critique from SNCC, the SCLC, or CORE would have elicited internal discussions and consideration of how to combat such a perception of the NAACP. By the late 1960s and early 1970s, Innis's comments caused no such reaction within the NAACP. In addition to the overall perception of the NAACP's preeminence within the movement, CORE, like SNCC, was organizationally weak at this time.[12] The NAACP did not perceive the declining radical organizations to be threats to its position within the now-disintegrating movement.[13] The NAACP made its disdain for the goals of the militant organizations explicit in its response to the NUL call for a coalition of Black organizations:

> The experience of the NAACP with various attempts at unity has not been happy. In the present situation some intermeshing of efforts of organizations would be enormously helpful. What we are unable to see, however, is how valuable to such an intermeshing would be the organizations which already have declared their allegiance to an organized political doctrine opposed to the United States. . . . We of the NAACP have long been on record for unity in the pursuit of the common goals of all Negro Americans. And we continue to believe that only the people who believe in the reformation of America belong in such a conference. The others have given up on America, or else they have chased after golden calves devised to suit their individual ideas of salvation.[14]

As opposed to the radical and militant groups, the NUL maintained its organizational strength during this period. Since its 1968 New Thrust initiatives on community-building in low-income African American communities, the NUL was increasingly perceived as more militant than the NAACP in its programming, but also maintained a closer, and more allied, relationship with the Nixon administration than did the

NAACP.[15] However, the NAACP did not feel threatened by the League's new programming, particularly because the group did not consider such organizing its strategic or programmatic focus.

The NUL received federal support for its New Thrust initiatives beginning in 1971, and carried federal contracts to implement its programming with numerous federal departments and agencies, including the OEO and the Departments of Defense and Housing and Urban Development. The NAACP distinguished itself from the NUL through its disinterest in federal funding and public statements highlighting the importance of retaining organizational independence from the federal government. In 1972, Simeon Booker wrote in his *Jet Magazine* column in that the NAACP received financial assistance from the Nixon administration. The NAACP responded quickly, explaining that the organization had received two government contracts during the Nixon administration, but had never profited from a contract. The NAACP did not want its membership to believe that the organization sacrificed any of its independence because it received financial assistance from the Nixon administration. At the NAACP's annual membership meeting in 1972, Wilkins stated:

> We don't want our members and supporters to get the idea that the Nixon Administration can be called on upon by the NAACP for "financial assistance." . . . It costs roughly $130,000 a month to run the NAACP. If we get into trouble, we will call up our members and contributors, not upon political candidates or parties.[16]

This statement reveals the NAACP's distinctiveness from NUL—it was a membership organization that did not receive federal government funding. Therefore, the NAACP did not consider its own position among civil rights groups to be threatened by the NUL.

The NAACP role within the civil rights niche was safe during the late 1960s and early 1970s. The more radical groups were losing public support, no longer competing for the support of white liberals, and no longer attempting to affect social change from within the system. Even the NUL began to embrace more rhetorically radical tactics, while at the same time receiving federal funding for its programming. Because of the struggles of other organizations, the NAACP had no need to worry that it would lose its place as the preeminent civil rights organization. The NAACP shift away from its antipoverty priorities emphasizes the importance of organizational competition to a group's priorities. The lack of competition for its constituency from other groups allowed the NAACP to return to its traditional priorities and tactics, rather than adjust its priorities based on the activities of other groups.

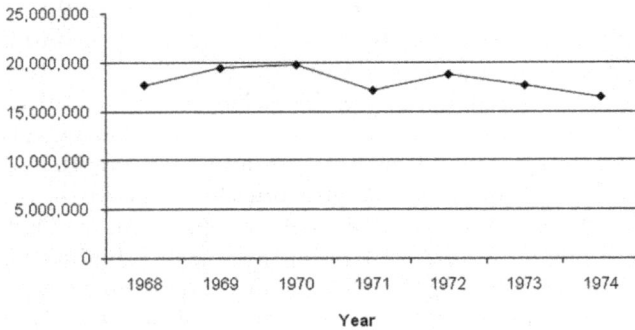

Figure 6.1. NAACP adjusted income, 1968–1974.

Trends in NAACP Growth

During the late 1960s and early 1970s, the NAACP struggled financially, although not to the same extent as other civil rights organizations. In 1970, the organization's annual report stated that members who left the organization during the mid-1960s were returning, after realizing that the NAACP was the most effective organization for fighting racism.[17] At the 1972 Convention, the national board compared the organization's financial health to that of other civil rights groups:

> At a time when several sister organizations reel in disarray, are in complete dissolution or have been diverted in their purposes, it is not by accident that the NAACP has been able to bring both stability and energy to its task. Two things have been primarily responsible for the growth and strength of this most broadly based and most widely feared and respected of the Civil Rights organizations: executive leadership and sound policy.[18]

Despite public statements of organizational health, the NAACP did experience declines in its income, membership, and branches during the late 1960s and early 1970s. As Figure 6.1 illustrates, the NAACP's income declined between 1970 and 1971, increased between 1971 and 1972, but then declined again between 1972 and 1974. During these periods of decline in income, Wilkins emphasized the importance of building the organization's membership. Although the NAACP did receive funding from foundations during this period, it continued to emphasize the importance of membership donations to the organization's health.[19] Upon receipt of a $300,000 grant from the Ford Foundation, Wilkins indicated that the organization could not rely on such assistance, and that membership was critical to its survival.[20]

Membership drives were particularly necessary during this period

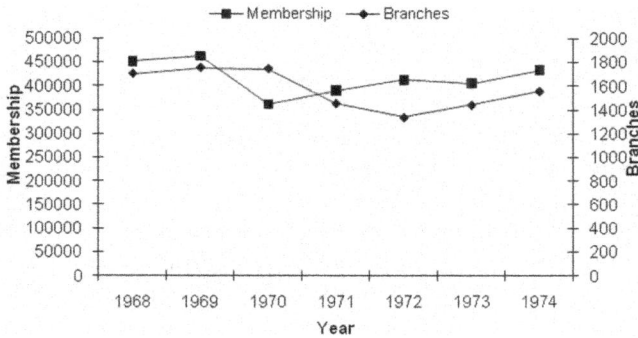

Figure 6.2. NAACP membership and branches, 1968–1974.

because, beginning in 1969, the national office began to increase membership fees.[21] The NAACP raised them from $2 to $4 in 1970 and to $5 in 1971. The organization had raised its membership fee only once before—in 1911 it was $1 per year.[22] Because of these increases, the national office focused on pushing branches to organize membership drives to fight the inevitable decline in membership upon fee hikes.[23] As Figure 6.2 indicates, the NAACP faced a substantial drop in membership after its fee increase in 1970. After the initial drop, the organization was able to increase its membership through drives, with the exception of a small drop between 1972 and 1973. By 1974, neither membership nor income had returned to its 1969 levels.

The number of NAACP branches also faced a substantial drop between 1970 and 1972—403 branches, or 23 percent of the organization's branches in 1970, were closed by 1972 (see Figure 6.2). This was the first year the number of branches declined since 1960, when the organization closed 95, or 10 percent, of its branches that were open in 1959. Branches were not the only NAACP entities facing closures during the early 1970s—because of financial difficulty, the NAACP closed seven regional training centers in 1972.[24]

During the War on Poverty, the NAACP stepped outside of its traditional strategies and activities to mobilize the poor at the local level. Such expansion was not attractive during the late 1960s and early 1970s, a period of financial difficulty for the NAACP. Instead, it returned to its more traditional strategies and programming. The organization focused on shoring up and maintaining its traditional constituencies, and on legal and legislative battles concerning employment nondiscrimination and housing. The NAACP Washington Bureau, led by Clarence Mitchell, was active concerning judicial appointments and legislation, and took a leadership role among civil rights organizations. The Bureau tracked legislation, such as the FAP, and offered testimony before congressional committees on other legislation of concern to the organization.[25] The NAACP did address anti-poverty policy through the Washington Bureau. However, it no longer engaged in nationally directed mobilizing activities on behalf of low-income African Americans. Its attention to national anti-poverty policy declined because the national office did not consider advocacy on behalf of the poor to be necessary to maintain its constituency, or its preeminence, as it had during the earlier period.

Factors Contributing to Declining NUL Attention to National Anti-Poverty Policy (1968-1972)

As I discuss in Chapter 4, NUL attention to anti-poverty policy, as measured by the organization's attention to the FAP, decreased between the late 1960s and early 1970s. By the early 1970s this attention had dropped to 47 percent of its level during the 1960s (see Table 6.1). The League's declining attention to national policy was due to its recommitment to social service delivery—the organization's founding purpose.

Beginning in 1968, the League's goals and priorities, and its structure, were determined by its New Thrust Initiative. Largely funded by foundations, the New Thrust re-focused NUL social service activities on low-income African American communities.[26]

> The burning and looting that have ravaged our cities are due in large measure to the unanswered cry from the people of the ghetto for a fair shake in becoming part of the larger American society. The Urban League must heed that cry with a renewed effort to turn its own resources, and indeed the resources and concern of all America, to that all-important task. . . . This new thrust recognizes our contributions of the past while addressing itself to the challenges of the present and opportunities for larger service in the future.[27]

Although the League had been providing social services to the poor since its founding, the New Thrust made anti-poverty services the primary NUL focus. To facilitate this shift in constituency, the national office increased its responsibility for the coordination of the activities of its affiliates: "Giving a voice to the voiceless, power to the powerlessness and pride and self-respect to the down-trodden are the ends toward which the UL is going to apply a dramatically increased effort. . . . Through community organization, the UL will help the ghetto free itself."[28] The New Thrust's nationally directed, and yet locally programmed, structure was attractive to the Nixon administration, which was searching for alternatives to the War on Poverty programs. In 1970, Whitney Young approached the administration to provide federal funding for the initiatives. Beginning in 1971, the Federal Thrust initiatives were funded by numerous federal agencies and departments.

Ironically, during the period when the NUL was wholly focused on programming to benefit low-income African Americans, the organization's level of attention to anti-poverty policy declined. During the New Thrust and Federal Thrust initiatives, the NUL was not focusing on national-level activities, as it had been during the War on Poverty. Instead, the national office increased its oversight and control over local affiliates, and supported grassroots programming by local offices—the national office did not require that local offices work to support national programming. As opposed to during the War on Poverty, the NUL's activities concerning anti-poverty legislation were almost wholly carried out by the Washington office. The external political environment led the League to determine that it must step away from national-level advocacy on behalf of the poor—its founding mission and internal structure determined its focus on social service provision for the poor during the late 1960s and early 1970s.

A Turn to Local Social Provision: The New and Federal Thrusts

By the late 1960s, civil rights organizations were functioning in a very different political climate than during the War on Poverty: Nixon was in the White House, the Vietnam War was the focus of white liberal activism, and the uprisings in American cities made the public and policymakers question the benefits of the civil and voting rights legislation. Similar to some national policymakers, the League increasingly believed that local attention was required to address, or quell, the distress in low-income African American areas. However, the NUL also increased its focus on the local level in response to the changing national political climate. In its report to the Ford Foundation after one year of the foundation's funding of the New Thrust initiative, the NUL explained its basis for changing its goals and priorities: "It was against the background . . . of increasing white intransigence, of growing black-white polarization, and of government retreat that the Urban League, early in 1968, began to prepare a blueprint for a new focus and direction to be known as New Thrust."[29] This new focus required a new conception of organizational goals and strategies:

> New Thrust, in effect, embodied a philosophical departure from many of the traditional Urban League goals, strategies, and roles which had determined its actions in the past. Instead of continuing in the role of power

broker between blacks and the white establishment, it determined to align itself much more closely to the black ghetto community, building new ties and new bases of operation within the ghetto as basic determinants of Urban League action.[30]

During 1968 and 1969, the New Thrust initiatives were funded primarily by foundations; in 1970, the NUL approached the Nixon administration to fund the programming.[31] Despite its frequent criticisms of the administration's proposed policies, the League had established a relationship with the White House, and was often consulted by officials on policies of interest to the League.[32] In August 1969, Young indicated that he had not yet written off the Nixon administration: "I am disappointed in the order of priorities and I am disappointed in the programs cut back and replaced. Mr. Nixon is intelligent and sensitive and I believe be wants to be president over a unified country."[33] Young's defense of the Nixon administration garnered national attention when he disagreed with NAACP president Bishop Spottswood, in his statements that Nixon was "anti-Negro." In response, Young stated that Nixon was not consciously anti-black, but that administration policies had negatively affected African Americans.[34]

On December 22, 1970, Young and other League officials met with President Nixon and secretaries of Agriculture, Commerce, Labor, HEW, HUD, Transportation, and with officials from the OEO and the Department of Defense. Young proposed that the Nixon administration begin to take advantage of groups, like the League, that had specific experience with human relations. Young proposed that federal programming be channeled through private agencies with an existing presence in black communities, such as the League.[35] Nixon agreed, and asked that each department secretary and agency director look into programming that would complement the League's work (Dickerson 1998, 266).

> Mr. Young complained that, whereas the government often lets our contracts to the private sector for the provision of military hardware and other manufactured goods, few such relationships exists in the private, non-profit, "software" industries . . . , which cater to human needs. In response, the President committed himself and his associates to a relationship with the League that would obligate the Federal Government to make sizeable outlays in the form of contracts to the League.[36]

The League submitted proposals for programs such as day care, family planning, and minority employment to the administrative agencies and departments. By January 1971, the organization was receiving federal funding for its proposed programs.[37] During 1971 and 1972, the NUL received $21.24 million in contracts from eight federal departments to implement programs supporting the goals of the New Thrust (Dickerson 1998, 266).

The League was aware of the concerns that such a close relationship with the federal government might evoke among its members and staff, and explicitly countered any suggestions that the NUL was becoming a "junior partner" to the federal government.[38] In his report to the 1971 Delegate Assembly, Harold Sims, acting executive director, weighed such concerns against the benefits of the federal funding:

> For the long term, while we are highly conscious of our need to preserve our freedom of action in our relationship with the public sector, we also view the prospect of increased access to federal funds as a great opportunity to provide services of all sorts in new areas where, for lack of money, such expansion was not possible before.[39]

Vernon Jordan, executive director designate, explicitly addressed concerns that the Federal Thrust programming would squelch NUL critiques of the Nixon administration at the same Delegate Assembly. He reassured the delegates that NUL would continue to criticize the Nixon administration when its actions warranted critique:

> We will pursue our joint ventures with the government without abdicating our right to disagree when the occasion warrants disagreement. . . . We have been in business for over 60 years without appreciable federally financed programs in the past, and we have now undertaken those commitments not out of an institutional urge to expand, but out of a sense of dedication to the cause of all black and minority people, and by extension, to the cause of building a prouder and better America.[40]

By 1972, the NUL was a very different organization than it had been during 1968. Its programs were largely federally funded, and the national office was engaged in local-level organizing, as well as social service provision. The Federal Thrust allowed the organization to expand in terms of income and affiliates during a period when many civil rights organizations were in a state of decline, contributing to the League's devotion of its resources to advocacy on behalf of the poor. As Figure 6.3 illustrates, the organization's income and chapters increased steadily between 1967 and 1973, with a slight decline in income between 1970 and 1971. Although the League increased its social service provision to the poor during this period, the organization's structural changes also led it to decrease its attention to anti-poverty policy at the national level.

NUL Structural Changes: Increased National Direction of Affiliate Priorities

The NUL functioned as a federated organization for much of its history—local Leagues were autonomous organizations that determined

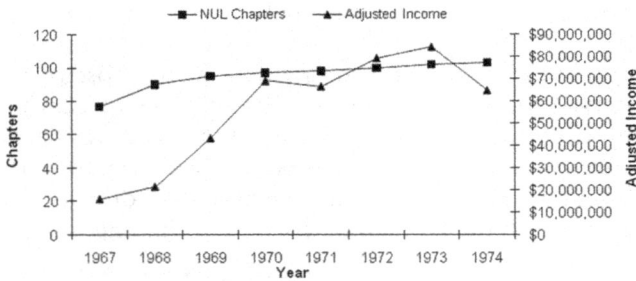

Figure 6.3. NUL adjusted income and chapters, 1967–1974. Income adjusted to 2002 dollars.

their own priorities and programming. During the War on Poverty, national oversight of affiliate activities increased—this oversight became institutionalized during the late 1960s and early 1970s. In 1968, the NUL received a Ford Foundation grant of over $1 million to "reorient the practices and policies of this organization's 90 affiliates" to the New Thrust activities.[41] The New Thrust initiatives were particularly challenging for local offices because they required new community-level programming by the local affiliates and increased oversight of this programming by the national office. In its 1969 application to the Ford Foundation for additional funding of New Thrust activities, the NUL pointed to the changing role of affiliates as the biggest challenge to implementation of New Thrust programs: "The traditional affiliate structure . . . had to be revamped into a problem-solving mechanism providing for active ghetto participation."[42] By 1969, tightening the relationship with local offices was the national office's top priority. Regional offices were created as arms to oversee and provide services to affiliates.

The national office distributed an operations manual to direct the affiliates in their implementation of New Thrust programs. The instructions were particularly important because many League affiliates were not already operating in low-income areas and were required to perform outreach activities, and in some cases to physically move, in order to achieve the goals of the New Thrust. The Manual indicated that affiliates should send a proposal to the Field Services Office in Washington outlining their own plans for implementation of New Thrust programming.[43] The national field staff would be responsible for researching national trends in social service provision, and for providing listings of community resources, local groups, and skilled local staff that may be helpful in the implementation of New Thrust initiatives.[44]

Despite its attempts to centralize priorities, the national office remained frustrated with the relationship between the national office and local affiliates by late 1970, just before the Nixon administration committed federal funding for the New Thrust initiatives. Because of these frustrations, the NUL cabinet, the organization's planning body, created the Central Planning Unit to coordinate the programming and strategies of the national office and local affiliates. At the meeting to create the unit, Sterling Tucker, a close advisor to Young and the executive director of the Washington Urban League, presented the NUL cabinet with the organization's major structural problems, and pointed to the programmatic disconnect between the national and local offices:

> [The first major national programming problem is] . . . the lack of a unified national program focus for the entire [NUL] movement—a focus predicated by an identifiable and accepted agency mission. The result is a national and local ambivalence in program content . . . there is a continued disparity in program priorities and content between national and locals as well as among the 97 affiliates.[45]

The significant influx of federal funding to the NUL during 1971 and 1972 made improved central planning more critical to the national office:

> The emergence of the Federal Thrust . . . makes . . . overall planning more imperative than ever and provides an ideal take-off point for developing comprehensive and integrated approaches and directions for the entire [NUL] movement. . . . The objectives, strategies, and program of all NUL components and local affiliates must be determined by this central mission and direction.[46]

Concerns about the relationship among NUL offices were not limited to the national level. In 1971, the executive directors of local leagues called the relationship between the national and local offices at a "grave level" of deterioration.[47] The local executive directors called for increased programmatic direction from the national office, pointing to a lack of a "common Urban League system" that would include the priorities and program objectives for all affiliates.[48] These frustrations of the local executive directors reflect the dual demands of the national office: that the local offices conduct their own grassroots campaigns while becoming less autonomous in terms of programming.

Attempts to tighten the relationship between the local and national offices were made League policy on July 28, 1971, when the Delegate Assembly adopted a revised Terms of Affiliation. The new terms increased national oversight of affiliate activities: the national office would provide each affiliate with an organizational manual outlining structure and procedure for all Leagues, ongoing consultation and support, and orientation and in-service training for affiliate staff. For the first time in NUL history, each affiliate would be evaluated periodically by the national office, and any failure to abide by the provisions laid out by the national office could result in probation, suspension, or disaffiliation.[49]

In addition to tightening the relationship between the national and local offices, the national office considered particular structural changes within the League to be necessary to build an institutional relationship between the League and the federal government: "With the emergence of the federal resources program, the Washington arm of the NUL must be prepared to take on immense new responsibilities as the liaison with the federal establishment."[50] After Whitney Young's death in March 1971, Sterling Tucker wrote to Harold Sims, the acting executive director, explaining that the infusion of federal funds would require the NUL to engage in organizational expansion: "today we are a different organization than we were three months ago, before the federal resources came upon the scene."[51]

To better fulfill its new role with the federal government, the duties of the Washington Bureau were expanded and it was renamed the Department of Governmental Affairs in 1971. After six months of operation, the Department reported that its activities included monitoring the Congressional Record and hearings, providing written and oral testimony on issues of concern to the league, working with administrative offices, and providing leadership in civil rights coalitions.[52] The Department was responsible for keeping the New York national office up to date on legislative issues, as well as providing documents on national priorities to regional offices and local affiliates.

By 1971, the League's resources had been almost wholly devoted to New Thrust programming for two years. "In the last two years, the tenets of New Thrust—community organization, institutional change, grassroots orientation, problem solving—have attained an undisputed priority position in the Urban League's philosophical scheme."[53] The singular focus on the New and Federal Thrusts, and hence on improving the relationship between the national and local organizations, did not leave time or resources for a high level of organizational attention to the FAP. Attention to the policy was left to the Department of Government Affairs and did not become an organization-wide priority. In the case of the NUL, the tightening of the relationship between the national and local offices was for the purpose of improving services for the poor, but did not lead to increased policy advocacy on behalf of them. The NUL was focusing on work within communities, and on strengthening affiliate presence in low-income African American areas.

During the early 1970s, the League retained its commitment to political activity, and expanded the scope of the Washington office. Although the Department of Government Affairs was active concerning legislation, the national office devoted itself to helping affiliates organize their communities. The New Thrust initiatives increased local League organizing in low-income African American communities; once the federal government began to fund those initiatives, it became imperative to the national office that it increase its oversight of affiliate programming and organizing. It was not a lack of national office activities that led to its decline in attention in anti-poverty activities; rather, it was that affiliates and local offices were not receiving instructions about participating in national level anti-poverty activities. Because of changes in the political environment, and external funding, the League underwent internal changes that led the national office to reprioritize national level anti-poverty activities in favor of community organizing.

Conclusions

Although both the NAACP and the NUL decreased their levels of attention to anti-poverty policy during the late 1960s and early 1970s, they did so very different reasons. The NAACP no longer had an incentive to move beyond its traditional strategies and constituency. The NUL's decreased attention, on the other hand, was based on its increased commitment to local grassroots organizing in low-income African American communities. Despite these differences, the NUL and NAACP cases shed light on the factors that lead groups to shift their priorities. Both cases point to the importance of the interaction between internal and external factors in the determination of organizational priorities. For the NAACP, changes in the civil rights issue niche, and organizational financial difficulties, led the organization to decrease its attention to anti-poverty policy. For the NUL, changes in the political and economic environments led the organization to rethink its mission and strategies, and to eventually decrease its national anti-poverty advocacy.

The late 1960s and early 1970s was a period of redefinition for the civil rights issue niche. Despite changes, the dynamics among organizations continued to affect organizational priorities, particularly for the NAACP. The case studies of organizational behavior during the 1970s extend my findings beyond the perhaps exceptional case of the civil rights movement of the 1960s. Even as coordination among civil rights organizations, and the number of groups, declined, organizational priorities were determined by the activities of organizations with similar missions. The NUL's uniqueness within the issue niche led it to engage in a restructuring to capture federal dollars for community organizing; the NAACP's regained preeminence within the niche allowed it to resume its traditional goals and strategies.

Chapter 7

Recent Battles, Recent Challenges

---

a . . . devastating hurricane strikes New Orleans. Neither the President nor any other federal official is there to help. . . . Thousands [were] stranded and they [were] overwhelmingly black and poor. That was horrendous enough. Even worse was that it [took] five days before meaningful help [arrived]. Some would say . . . that we witnessed a modern-day lynching.
  —Julian Bond, Chairman of the NAACP National Board of Directors

[The National Urban League has] occasionally [been] accused of being a middle class organization. I used to say that if the charge is that our goal is to help poor people get into the middle class, we are guilty with gusto.
  —Hugh B. Price, President and CEO of the National Urban League

Civil rights organizations varied in their responses to the needs of the poor during two recent, and different, policy battles—welfare reform during the mid-1990s and the response to Hurricane Katrina between 2005 and 2008. Drawing on organizational documents and interviews with leaders and staff, I assess NAACP and NUL attention to issues of poverty during each period. Since organizational archives are not yet available for such recent times, I largely rely on public documents and media coverage of events and activities, neither of which provide an understanding of *why* groups chose to address particular issues at different times.[1] Therefore, I assess how much attention groups devoted to anti-poverty issues, using lessons from my research on earlier periods to discuss why groups varied their attention to issues affecting low-income

African Americans—an important first step in understanding representation of the poor in the U.S. political system.

Although the universe of civil rights organizations has unquestionably changed, and possibly shrunk, over the past forty years, such groups remain vitally important for the political representation of African Americans at the local and national levels. How have such organizations responded in recent years when the interests of low-income African Americans are being addressed, and sometimes threatened, by government? Like other welfare reform policies analyzed in earlier chapters, those debated during the 1990s sought to overhaul the system; indeed, they were considered to be the most significant set of reforms since the War on Poverty. Although the catastrophe of Hurricane Katrina is clearly not a matter of welfare policy alone, the sudden national attention to race and poverty presented advocacy organizations with a unique opportunity. Any analysis of advocacy on behalf of low-income African Americans would be remiss if it neglected such a significant moment in recent history.

My findings indicate that the NAACP and NUL varied in the levels of attention they devoted to issues affecting low-income African Americans during the mid-1990s and in response to Katrina, but that neither organization devoted a high level of attention to such activities. Groups were struggling financially, and working primarily on issues of employment discrimination and affirmative action. Overall, the voices of the poor were notably absent during the reform battles of the mid-1990s—no radical group primarily concerned with civil rights issues was active enough to push civil rights organizations to advocate on behalf of low-income African Americans.[2]

On the other hand, civil rights organizations devoted substantial attention to Hurricane Katrina. As Figure 7.1 reflects, they organized donation drives, raised the issue of poverty through their publications, and advocated for the poor in state capitals and on Capitol Hill. The Urban League credited Katrina with turning the organization's attention back to one of its founding missions, to advocate economic equality for African Americans. However, as Katrina lost the media spotlight and the nation's attention turned elsewhere, so did that of civil rights organizations. After their initial response, the NAACP and NUL did less in terms of policy follow-through. Without a mass-based, national focus on the poor, mainstream groups no longer felt incentives to increase their own advocacy.

I begin the next section with a discussion of the organizational response to welfare reform during the mid-1990s. Both the NAACP and NUL responded to welfare reform during two periods: 1995 and 1996, when the plan was being debated in Congress and eventually passed;

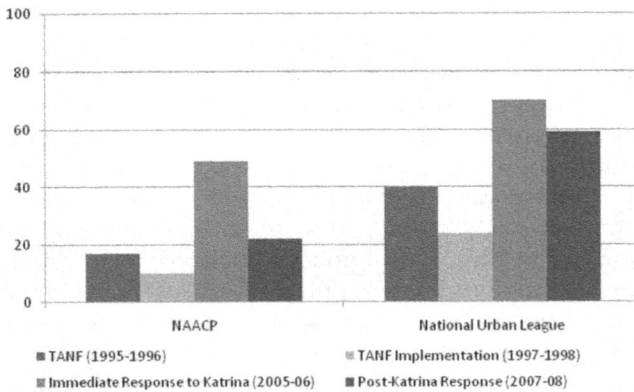

Figure 7.1. NAACP and NUL response to TANF and Hurricane Katrina.

and 1997 and 1998, when advocacy groups responded to welfare reform's passage and plans for implementation. Second, I present the strong civil rights advocacy response to Hurricane Katrina in 2005 and 2006 and the weakening response during 2007 and 2008. I assess the levels of attention each organization devoted to issues affecting low-income African Americans during these periods and discuss possible reasons for their shifting levels of attention.

Reforming the Welfare System (1995–1998)

Both the Democratic and Republican parties emphasized the need to reform welfare in the 1994 congressional elections and again in the 1996 presidential election. Welfare reform was included in the Republicans' *Contract with America,* and Democratic presidential nominee Bill Clinton campaigned on a promise to "End welfare as we know it"—a promise that would be realized when he signed the Personal Responsibility and Work Opportunity Reconciliation Act (PRWORA) of 1996. Policymakers expressed concern about the "dependence" of welfare recipients on the system, and a lack of work requirements for those receiving aid. In addition to these explicit goals, the proposed policy attempted to legislate federal government support for a traditional, male-led family structure.[3] The 1996 reforms were presented as the most sweeping reforms in the history of welfare in the United States, ending the entitlement programs encompassed in the AFDC program. During debates on the legislation, advocates and scholars were concerned with the effects of reform on the

African American poor, particularly if a jobs program was not included along with the cuts to welfare spending.[4]

The effort to pass welfare reform legislation was bipartisan, but differences between the parties arose in regard to specific requirements in the legislation. Democrats opposed particular provisions in the initial Republican-sponsored legislation in Congress, such as the time limits based on work requirements, the ineligibility of legal immigrants, and the failure to include a national jobs program. However, Clinton's promise to "End welfare as we know it" required him to focus on welfare reform, and eventually to sign a bill that included provisions that the administration opposed. The notion that the system must be reformed trumped concern about specific provisions of that reform.[5] Because of a sense of urgency to reform welfare, many opponents of provisions within the legislation were willing to compromise. Nonetheless, the inclusion of work requirements coupled with the legislation's failure to include a jobs program led to three resignations within the Clinton administration, including that of Peter Edelman in the Department of Health and Human Services (Smith 2007, 253). The NAACP and NUL were unwavering in their opposition to the legislation, particularly because of the inclusion of work requirements without a federal jobs program.[6]

The NAACP Response to Welfare Reform

The mid- to late 1990s were a difficult period for the NAACP both organizationally and financially. By 1996, the national office was in debt for millions of dollars and headed toward bankruptcy. Affiliates reported that they were close to closing their doors and fully dependent on donations members sent through the mail.[7] Most of the organization's activities were curtailed during this period, even those concerning traditional priorities such as affirmative action.

As Table 7.1 reflects, the NAACP did not devote substantial attention to Temporary Aid to Needy Families (TANF) reform, although it did offer analysis of the legislation as President Clinton's version was being compared to the Republicans'. An article in *The Crisis* compared the two plans and concluded that analysts concerned with issues of poverty and welfare were supporting Clinton's plan, despite earlier reservations:

> Clinton introduced a welfare reform bill in Congress to change the public assistance system. . . . Republican members of Congress included a set of more stringent proposals for welfare reform in September. . . . Many analysts had serious reservations about the Clinton plan. But it now looks good [to them] in comparison to the Republican proposal. Whichever plan wins, welfare reform of some sort seems to be inevitable. The only question is

Table 7.1. NAACP Attention to Welfare Reform (TANF) and Hurricane Katrina

Organizational activities	TANF reform (1994–1996)	TANF implementation (1997–1998)	Immediate response to Katrina (2005–2006)	Follow-up to Katrina (2007–2008)
Low priority indicators (1 point each)				
• Position taken on issue (statement, convention resolution)	X	X	X	X
Mid-level priority indicators (2 points each)				
• Staff, or organizational committee, assigned to issue as one of several, or only, assignments	X			
• Internal evidence of funding for activities concerning issue	n/a	n/a	n/a	n/a
• Communications to policy-makers about issue (testimonies before Congress or parties, position letters)			X	X
• Public speeches or statements by staff/leadership about issue	X	X	X	
• National Office directs local branches/affiliates to be active on issue	X		X	X
• Mailings to membership about issue	n/a	n/a	X	

High-level priority indicators (3 points each)	17%	10%	49%	22%
• Fundraising with membership about issue				
• Mobilization of membership for actions about issue			X	X
• Consultation with policy-makers about issue (legislative drafting, implementation)				X
• National office offers workshops/training for local branches/affiliates on issue				
• Internal discussions indicate issue as priority	n/a	n/a	X	
• Organizational documents name the issue as a priority (resolutions, annual reports, org. publications)				
• Organizational restructuring to address issue (overall restructuring, creation of new department)				
• Organization offers own plan concerning issue				
No evidence of priority				
• Absence of any evidence of issue as priority				
Priority level	17%	10%	49%	22%

*Priority level determined by organization activities as percentage of total possible activities. NAACP activities during 1994–1996 totaled 5 of 30 possible points, a 17% priority score; 1997–1998 totaled 3 of 30 possible points, a 10% priority score; 2005–2006 totaled 18 of 37 possible points, a 49% priority score; 2007–2008 totaled 8 of 37 possible points, a 22% priority score.

how punitive it will be and what impact it will have on the lives of those who must endure it.[8]

In addition to providing such analysis, the NAACP participated in coalitions with other concerned interest groups offering response to the legislation.[9] As unemployment and homelessness increased throughout American cities, the organization devoted attention to issues of poverty beyond welfare reform. The NAACP dedicated its final issue of *The Crisis* in 1995 to the issue of homelessness.[10]

Although the national office was relatively inactive on welfare reform, affiliates indicated that they were tracking the legislative proposals, especially after the inclusion of TANF reform in the 1994 *Contract with America*.[11] When Myrlie Evers-Williams took over as NAACP Chairman of the Board in 1995, she named welfare reform as one of the issues the organization would watch most closely in Congress.[12] Despite Evers-Williams's intentions, the national office did not engage in activity concerning the proposed legislation. At the organization's 1997 annual meeting, Executive Director Kweisi Mfume explained the organization's silence on issues considered to be relevant to the group: "This organization was almost at the cliff's edge. . . . There was and there still remains a lot of question about the relevancy of the association."[13] Although Mfume spent his first year working to rebuild the NAACP internally, he indicated that the group would soon return to its traditional priorities, including welfare reform.[14] In his explanation of the future plans of the organization, he stated that "The NAACP will take the lead in defending affirmative action, shaping welfare reform, teaching tolerance."[15] Such promises reflected the organization's inactivity during the mid-1990s. Due to its severe organizational and financial difficulties the NAACP was unable to pursue many of its traditional priorities, let alone offer substantial advocacy on an issue that was often low on the organization's priority list.

The NUL Response to Welfare Reform

Consistently concerned about issues of poverty and economic opportunity for African Americans, the NUL devoted attention to welfare as it was debated in 1995 and 1996, as Table 7.2 shows. Although the focus on economic issues was not a new one for the League, the organization had recently reconsidered its primary purpose and refocused its attention on policies that "would move African Americans into the economic mainstream."[16] In the 1995 *State of Black America*, the League's yearly publication, the organization reflected on its renewed emphasis on eco-

Table 7.2. NUL Attention to Welfare Reform (TANF) and Hurricane Katrina

Organizational activities	TANF reform (1994–1996)	TANF implementation (1997–1998)	Immediate response to Katrina (2005–2006)	Follow-up to Katrina (2007–2008)
Low-priority indicators (1 point each)				
• Position taken on issue (statement, convention resolution)	X	X	X	X
Mid-level priority indicators (2 points each)				
• Staff, or organizational committee, assigned to issue as one of several, or only, assignments	X	X	X	X
• Internal evidence of funding for activities concerning issue	n/a	n/a	n/a	n/a
• Communications to policy-makers about issue (testimonies before Congress or parties, position letters)	X	X	X	X
• Public speeches or statements by staff/leadership about issue	X	X	X	X
• National office directs local branches/affiliates to be active on issue	X		X	
• Mailings to membership about issue	n/a	n/a		X

Table 7.2. (Continued)

Organizational activities	TANF reform (1994–1996)	TANF implementation (1997–1998)	Immediate response to Katrina (2005–2006)	Follow-up to Katrina (2007–2008)
High-level priority indicators (3 points each)				
• Fundraising with membership about issue			X	
• Mobilization of membership for actions about issue			X	
• Consultation with policy-makers about issue (legislative drafting, implementation)	X	X	X	X
• National office offers workshops/training for local branches/affiliates on issue				
• Internal discussions indicate issue as priority	n/a	n/a	n/a	n/a
• Organizational documents name issue as a priority (resolutions, annual reports, org. publications)			X	
• Organizational restructuring to address issue (overall restructuring, creation of new department)				
• Organization offers own plan concerning issue			X	X
No evidence of priority				
• Absence of any evidence of issue as priority				
*Priority level**	40%	24%	70%	59%

*Priority level determined by organization activities as percentage of total possible activities. NUL activities during 1994–1996 totaled 12 of 30 possible points, a 40% priority score; 1997–1998 totaled 8 of 30 possible points, a 24% priority score; 2005–2006 totaled 26 of 37 possible points, a 70% priority score; War on Poverty period totaled 22 of 37 possible points, a 59% priority score.

nomic advancement and pointed out that this goal had been embraced
by the NUL since its founding:

> millions of our people remain stuck on the down escalator, headed
> nowhere or worse. Their dire circumstances must dwell in our consciences
> because of the tragic loss of human potential and the mounting drain on
> societal resources and compassion. It is their fate, then, that must be the
> primary focus of the Urban League movement. This renewed emphasis on
> our sisters and brothers and children in greatest need honors our original
> mission, which was to serve those of us in meager circumstances who are
> seeking access to mainstream society.[17]

Hugh B. Price, president and CEO, argues that such a restatement of
the organization's mission was necessary to distinguish it among other
organizations and to reflect its activities:

> The change in the mission statement was a bit of a shift. I wanted to engi-
> neer that shift in thinking because we were forever known as the "second
> oldest" and "second largest" civil rights organization. I kept saying as we
> approach the 100th anniversary, we'd better be known as the biggest and
> oldest . . . at something, rather than the second. The other reality is that in
> fact what the Urban League does nationally and at the local level is princi-
> pally about helping people make that journey into the [economic] main-
> stream . . . if you look at the driving activity at the ground level and at the
> national level it's about the policy and programs that help people make
> the journey from poverty to the mainstream.[18]

To address the issues facing disadvantaged African Americans, the
League explained that it must focus specifically on particular approaches due to its limited resources. Price named three areas of focus:
education of children growing up in the inner-city, economic self-
sufficiency for their families, and racial inclusion so that African Americans could fully participate in the economy.[19] Consistent with the
League approach to economic development for African Americans,
public assistance policy was not specifically named as one of its areas of
focus.

Despite this decision, the Urban League continued to be active concerning welfare reform during the mid-1990s. Working with a coalition
of organizations including the Children's Defense Fund, the National
Council of La Raza, and the Joint Center for Political and Economic
Studies, the League advocated a welfare reform policy that would
include time limits and work requirements as qualifications for welfare
receipt, and a job creation program:

> We were alarmed because the welfare reform that [Clinton] endorsed . . .
> was basically a two-sentence welfare reform plan, and they dropped the
> second sentence. The first sentence was "you shouldn't live on welfare and

there will be time limits." But also there was the expectation that there
would be some type of employment program to help people move into the
private sector . . . that second sentence was dropped.[20]

The implications of decisions not to devote resources to anti-poverty
work during the debates over welfare policy raised concerns that programs intended to help the poor were too expensive. The League
addressed these implications, pointing out that they made the proposed
jobs program seem increasingly unlikely.

> Can society afford a jobs program for the poor? Let me pose the question
> a different way. Can we afford all the homelessness and anger that will
> result if mothers and children, cut off of welfare and without work, land
> on the streets?[21]

The League was very concerned that if the economy softened as compared to its relative strength during the mid-1990s and jobs disappeared,
individuals unable to find employment would be ineligible for welfare
benefits because of time limits.[22] As the final reform legislation made its
way to President Clinton's desk, the Urban League encouraged him to
veto it.[23] Price explained his understanding of congressional plans: "It
appears that Congress has wearied of the 'War on Poverty' and switched
sides and decided to wage war against poor people instead."[24]

After the passage of the 1996 welfare reform plan, the NUL worked
with the Department of Housing and Urban Development on economic
and community empowerment programs. In its 1997 annual report, the
League explained that the provisions in the welfare reform plan necessitated such work: "The loss of jobs and the reality of welfare reform
require innovative solutions and partnerships between federal, state and
local governments, and public and non-profit institutions."[25] In fact, the
NUL worked closely with HUD field staff to implement HUD-sponsored
and related programs in the areas of housing and economic development. It explained that such a partnership drew on the organization's
initial mission and purpose: "In finding solutions to the employment,
housing and basic services needs of the urban poor, the partnership with
HUD helps the Urban League continue the tradition established by its
founders at the beginning of the century."[26]

As Figure 7.1 reflects, the League considered welfare to be a part of
its newly-reconceived mission to help low-income African Americans
join in the economic mainstream. Because of the League's redefinition
of its purpose—implemented to distinguish it from other civil rights
organizations—welfare reform proposals necessitated organizational
attention, despite the ongoing NUL financial constraints. Once the legislation passed without a jobs program, the NUL continued to work with

the federal government on implementation, but turned its strongest attention to pressing priorities such as education reform.

Advocacy Response to an Unnatural Disaster: Hurricane Katrina and Its Aftermath

Hurricane Katrina made landfall in New Orleans on Monday, August 29, 2005, as a Category 4 hurricane. The George W. Bush administration had declared a federal state of emergency in Louisiana two days earlier, giving the Department of Homeland Security (DHS) and the Federal Emergency Management Agency (FEMA) the authority to respond. On Sunday, August 28, New Orleans Mayor Ray Nagin issued an unprecedented mandatory evacuation of the city. By late that afternoon, there were reports that water was beginning to breach levees, and New Orleans residents were gathering at the Superdome. On Wednesday, August 31, National Guard troops arrived, and President Bush organized a task force to coordinate the minimal federal response as he toured New Orleans without deplaning from Air Force One. Conditions in the Superdome soon became dangerous and unsanitary. Evacuees had no access to water, food, medical assistance, or bathroom facilities. National media were reporting rapes and deaths within the Superdome. Mayor Nagin and Louisiana Governor Kathleen Bianco made repeated requests for federal assistance, but remained desperate and frustrated while the federal government began to critique the state and local response. Throughout this period, the American public watched images of New Orleans residents who were stranded and struggling to survive.[27]

Katrina and its aftermath brought issues of race and poverty, and the intersection of the two, into the national spotlight. As a member of the staff at a civil rights organization explains:

> It's not fashionable to talk about "poverty" today or even to use the word "poor." Until Hurricane Katrina reminded the nation that poverty still existed and the poor are still with us, poverty and poor people hadn't been talked about for nearly 40 years at the national level.

It was not surprising that those who were trapped within the city were primarily poor and African American, since low-income African Americans made up 70 percent of the city's population.[28] Nor was it surprising that the response to Katrina sparked a debate about the appropriate relationship among the federal, state, and local governments. Federal attention and assistance to cities had been weak for some time (Dreier 2006). As Strolovitch, Warren, and Frymer argue in their analysis for the Social Science Research Council: "Race has always been central to debates about the proper role of the American government in aiding those Americans in need of assistance from the inequalities that result directly from the actions of both the government and private citizens."[29]

Civil rights organizations, including the NAACP and the NUL, recognized that advocacy on behalf of low-income African Americans in New Orleans was desperately necessary and that Katrina offered a unique opportunity to engage the broader American public in a conversation about race and poverty. These and other organizations were involved in advocacy on behalf of New Orleans residents even before the hurricane made landfall, lobbying the administration and Congress for appropriations. As the crisis continued, groups pushed for governmental restructuring to ensure that such an inadequate response could not occur again even as they pushed for housing and income assistance for displaced residents and tax incentives for business relocation in affected areas.[30]

As others have pointed out, however, national attention to issues of race and poverty in the aftermath of Katrina was relatively short-lived.[31] Despite media coverage immediately following the hurricane that documented its disproportionate impact on African Americans, white Americans were generally unwilling to connect the federal government's faulty response to the hurricane to the race of the victims. Although 60 percent of African Americans attributed the federal response to Katrina to the fact that the victims were African American, only 12 percent of whites agreed.[32] As national attention to the crisis faded, so did that of civil rights organizations; throughout 2007 and 2008 both NAACP and NUL maintained attention to the inadequacy of the federal response, although not at the same levels as immediately following Katrina.

The NAACP's Immediate Response to Katrina (2005–2006)

The NAACP named Katrina as a priority during 2005 and 2006. As Table 7.1 reflects, the organization opened satellite offices in the Gulf region, filed lawsuits on behalf of residents of the Gulf Coast, coordinated affiliate activities, and ran national fund-raising campaigns. The NAACP claimed to be the first group to get aid and supplies into Mississippi. *The Crisis* highlighted its immediate activities in response to the hurricane:

> Bruce Gordon, president and CEO of the NAACP, visited the area immediately after holding a September 3 press conference. . . . "Until every life has been stabilized and every life saved, we will devote all of our energies to that purpose . . . let there be no question, we need to be vigilant."

While Gordon and others were headed toward the Gulf Coast, four vans carrying nearly 50 NAACP members from Jackson, MS and Atlanta also traveled to the area to provide relief to those who had lost everything.[33]

The 2005 annual report delineated the NAACP's strategy: "Providing immediate assistance, ensuring equitable distribution of federal, state, and local money and resources, and ensuring the equitable reconstruction of affected areas and families."[34] The organization aggressively raised money, established the NAACP Disaster Relief Fund, and explained to its members that it would devote some funds for immediate aid while setting aside a portion of the money raised for longer-term housing needs.

> The NAACP . . . began soliciting donations for a Disaster Relief Fund to assist survivors of the storm. . . . When it came time to decide what to do with the money, the civil rights organization had a strategic decision to make. . . . A senior leadership council decided that the organization would provide direct assistance grants for individuals, families and students with immediate needs. The council, however, also wanted to provide a more long-term solution to Katrina victims. . . . In February [2006] [NAACP and Habitat for Humanity] joined forces and resources to help victims in the Gulf region whose homes were damaged.[35]

Within days of the disaster the organization recruited celebrity Jamie Foxx to serve as the spokesperson for the Disaster Relief Fund and organized a visit from Foxx and the executive director of the Hollywood Bureau, Vic Bulluck, to the Houston Superdome. Foxx and Bulluck worked with affiliate members to distribute assistance.[36]

The NAACP national office worked with local affiliates as well as charitable organizations such as the American Red Cross, the Salvation Army, and UNICEF. It joined other civil rights organizations, including the NUL, the Rainbow/PUSH Coalition, the National Coalition on Black Civil Participation, and the Congressional Black Caucus, in a meeting with the Bush administration immediately after the hurricane. Coalition partners recognized that their responses to Katrina could not be short-lived, but rather would require long-term commitment.[37]

In addition to direct aid and recovery activities related to the hurricane, the NAACP addressed issues of poverty more generally. In the first issue of *The Crisis* in 2006, economist William E. Spriggs examined the increased attention to poverty issues brought on by Katrina, the need for public policy to address poverty, and the myth that African American women disproportionately have children out of wedlock. Discussing Katrina's impact on public opinion concerning the appropriate role for public policy in fighting poverty, Spriggs pointed out that in a change from earlier polls, the majority of respondents now believed that the government should be responsible for alleviating poverty.[38]

One year after the hurricane, the organization put the recovery efforts and NAACP activities on the front page of the *NAACP Advocate*, a publication of the research, advocacy, and training division within the national office. Throughout 2006, the organization focused on the failure of restoration of housing in the Gulf Coast, emphasizing the disproportionate impact of the housing crisis on low-income residents:

> Despite promises and the commitment of billions of aid dollars, the reinvigoration of the region remains unrealized largely due to the failure to restore adequate housing . . . the crisis in housing is borne by the region's poorest residents. . . . Low-wage workers and families across the region are disproportionately impacted because a lack of affordable housing pushes low-wage workers further from job sites.[39]

Additionally, *The Crisis* continued to report on Katrina and highlighted first-person accounts of the impact of Katrina on the poor.[40] At the 2006 national convention (the first since the hurricane), delegates passed a resolution calling for a formal apology to victims from President Bush and Congress, a declaration of urgency for recovery, and specific policies such as fast processing of loans to African American businesses, waivers for payments of student loans, and increased eligibility for Medicaid.[41]

The national office was also active concerning the municipal elections scheduled for April 22, 2006, in New Orleans. The NAACP urged Governor Kathleen Blanco and U.S. Attorney General Alberto Gonzalez to reschedule the elections until voters who had been displaced by Katrina could be located. After the NAACP request was denied, the organization set up 16 voter assistance centers in nine states, including Georgia, Texas, Mississippi, and Alabama. The centers distributed voter registration forms and absentee ballots. The NAACP also worked with People for the American Way and the Leadership Conference for Civil Rights to set up a voter hotline; helped to coordinate a march and protest in New Orleans on the voting issue; and arranged for transportation for voters to return to New Orleans on election day.[42]

The NAACP was active at the federal level, lobbying Congress to increase funding for comprehensive relief legislation for hurricane victims. The organization included such funding on its list of priorities for the 109th Congress and sent action alerts to its membership to support funding legislation.[43] Members were asked to request that their members of Congress support proposed legislation to establish a victim restoration fund, increase environmental protections, address health issues of victims, extend housing and community development grants, protect voting rights, and expand small business opportunities.[44] Although the NAACP did not succeed in achieving these policy priorities, the organization activated its membership and called for policy change.

Affiliate Activities

In addition to its own response to Katrina, the national office coordinated and encouraged extensive responses by affiliates. The November/December 2005 issue of *The Crisis* emphasized the importance of the NAACP's "network of state and local branches" to its "extensive disaster relief campaign."[45] Immediately following the hurricane, the national office appointed a National Director of Disaster Relief and a liaison to the American Red Cross. The organization coordinated volunteers, ran fund-raising efforts, and distributed aid and supplies through disaster relief centers throughout the Gulf Coast:

> The massive undertaking involves not only soliciting monetary donations through the command center—more than $1 million was raised by the end of September—but also collecting and distributing supplies, locating temporary housing for thousands of displaced Gulf Coast residents and communicating with other relief organizations.[46]

Articles in *The Crisis* also highlighted the work of the Mississippi State Conference and Baton Rouge affiliates and their responsiveness to the needs of residents. The Baton Rouge affiliate specifically addressed complaints of police misconduct in the aftermath of the hurricane. The branch reported that it had received fifty to seventy-five complaints during the two months after Katrina, brought these complaints to the attention of the police chief, and held a community forum to address these concerns.[47] Local branches also welcomed evacuees from New Orleans and held food and supply drives for hurricane victims.[48]

The president of the Mississippi State Conference, Derrick Johnson, made immediate contact with FEMA and the American Red Cross to set up recovery centers in African American communities throughout Mississippi. Johnson claimed that the hurricane had reinvigorated the NAACP and its membership:

> Despite the numerous problems that have surfaced in Hurricane Katrina's wake, Johnson says this country's worst national disaster in history has strengthened the NAACP. "We have found that our organization has become stronger because of this and it has allowed many members around the state to recognize the strength of the organization."[49]

In March 2006, the NAACP opened a New Orleans Katrina Relief Center. The purpose of the Center was "to address a number of issues confronting Louisiana and the Gulf Coast states of Alabama, Mississippi and eastern Texas, including education, voting rights, housing, criminal justice matters and employment."[50] The national office hoped that the establishment of a more permanent institution would help with ongoing problems faced by residents. The NAACP reported that the Center provided an opportunity for residents, who were largely being ignored by policymakers at all levels, to be heard through community forums.

NAACP affiliates and centers throughout the Gulf Coast emphasized the disproportionate impact of the housing crisis on low-income and minority populations, wrote reports analyzing conditions, and offered recommendations to "ensure that further reconstruction is faster, fairer, and more effective."[51] The Mississippi report explicitly reflected the frustrations of residents attempting to return to New Orleans and expressed concern that aid was not reaching those with the most need.

> the response by federal and state policymakers toward rebuilding has been slow and not reflective of key voices in the state . . . proposed rebuilding policies have the potential to shift resources meant for the most vulnerable communities to areas that do not serve low-income citizens.[52]

The report emphasized the importance of protecting the interests of the working poor and ensuring that federal resources intended for the poor were not being diverted to more privileged communities.

The NAACP's Ongoing Response to Katrina (2007–2008)

As time passed after Katrina, the NAACP focused a greater proportion of its attention on the federal response to the disaster. During this period, the organization's CEO, Bruce Gordon, resigned over disagreements with the Board, and financial difficulties forced the organization to downsize. The national office laid off seventy employees as part of a "right-sizing" process.[53] While the group remained active, it focused many of its activities on Washington, D.C., a change that reflected its more limited organizational resources.

In 2007, as Congress returned from its August recess with sixty days to pass the 2008 budget, the NAACP pushed for increased funds for recovery. Julian Bond, chair of the national board, stated:

> We are approaching a moment of truth. . . . In the next 60 days we'll find out if those politicians were telling the truth when they made all their campaign promises and speeches about helping people recover their lives and livelihoods, or if they were just taking advantage of the victims of Katrina for political gain.[54]

The national office sent an action alert to its members explaining that "The President's budget proposal does not provide adequate funding for many of the key programs that provide housing, education, and health care assistance in the region."[55] The organization made a similar call to Congress in 2008 when it urged the passage of an employment and rebuilding plan:

> We need to show the people of New Orleans and the entire Gulf Coast region that the American public has not forgotten them . . . legislation would provide federal money to employ a minimum of 100,000 Gulf Coast residents who would work on projects to rebuild, sustain, and develop the Gulf Coast region.[56]

In the presidential election of 2008, the first since Hurricane Katrina, the NAACP assessed the Republican and Democratic platforms in relation to "Rebuilding the gulf coast after Hurricane Katrina" among thirty-three topics that the organization designated as priorities.[57] Bond emphasized that Katrina drew national attention to the issue of poverty and inequality, and that the NAACP should respond to this new national attention. In order to offer an effective response, the organization would need to strengthen its own organizational structures, and be prepared to work with other organizations:

> Racial inequality is imbedded into the fabric of post-civil rights movement American society. . . . We must make strengthening our Branches and State Conferences a first priority, building membership where it is low and insisting on activism where Branches are moribund. We must expand our outreach to and collaboration with our coalition partners—the time has long passed when we were the only soldiers in this fight. We cannot and should not go it alone.[58]

The NAACP continued its criticisms of the Bush administration through 2008. As the 2009 budget was being debated, the organization issued an action alert opposing Bush's proposed budget because it would "eliminate and/or cripple many crucial domestic services and programs while benefitting the wealthiest Americans." The organization wrote to members asking that they write their representatives and senators, asking for "continued assistance for those whose lives were devastated by Hurricanes Katrina and Rita in 2005."[59]

The national office called on affiliates to communicate to Congress the ongoing challenges faced by hurricane survivors and the Gulf region. In May 2008, the president of the Mississippi State Conference testified before the U.S. House Subcommittee on Housing and Community Opportunity addressing "the challenges and problems that continue to plague Mississippi coastal residents impacted by Hurricane Katrina."[60] In its press release announcing the testimony, the national office mentioned the affiliate's 2008 report on the unmet needs of Mississippi residents affected by the hurricane, previewing national media attention to the neglect of low-income individuals in the distribution of aid in Mississippi. The national office continued to emphasize the ongoing suffering of those affected by Katrina as the 2008 hurricane season threatened evacuations.

> The NAACP reminds the nation not to forget those who have still not fully recovered from the devastation of Hurricanes Rita and Katrina . . . NAACP branches and state conferences continue to work hard to secure proper health care, legal representation, education and housing in the Gulf Coast.[61]

National Support of Affiliate Activities

The organization continued to emphasize the ongoing activities of its affiliates in the area through 2007 and 2008. In an April 2007 press release Dennis C. Hayes, interim president and CEO, explained the centrality of affiliate activities to the organization's response: "In continuing our commitment to assist Katrina victims in the recovery . . . we will push the policy agenda to restore individuals' lives through our Louisiana affiliates, who are the residents of the affected areas and have a vested interest in succeeding in that effort."[62] The national office explained that the Gulf Coast Advocacy Center had been enveloped into the Louisiana State Conference of NAACP Branches, and that the Louisiana Conference would participate in research and advocacy to address the ongoing needs of hurricane victims. *The Crisis* reported that the New Orleans branch was working to ensure adequate housing and medical facilities and help returning students make the transition back to school.[63]

Marking the second anniversary of the hurricane in August and September 2007, the national office emphasized the organization's ongoing work in the area. "The NAACP's local and regional branches are working hard to ensure proper health care, legal representation, education and housing in the Gulf Coast."[64] Affiliates partnered with the Red Cross and Habitat for Humanity, and marked the second anniversary of the hurricane with town hall meetings that discussed the recovery in Alabama, Louisiana, and Mississippi.

In the immediate aftermath of Katrina, the NAACP devoted its organizational resources to aiding victims, supporting affiliates, lobbying Congress and the White House, and raising funds among its membership. The NAACP anti-poverty activities during 2005 and 2006 were slightly less significant to the organization than such activities during the War on Poverty of the 1960s, but more so than during the Family Assistance Plan of the early 1970s. The organization recognized the importance of remaining relevant during the response to Katrina and encouraged local branches to work in coalition with other groups.

As national attention to Hurricane Katrina waned during 2007 and 2008, so did the NAACP's. The organization devoted less attention to outreach among its membership through fundraising and activism campaigns. Without the national media and political pressure, the NAACP returned to its more traditional priorities, such as housing and job discrimination, while continuing to monitor the federal government's response to Katrina.

The NUL's Immediate Response to Hurricane Katrina

The NUL made its response to Katrina a top priority during the period immediately following the hurricane. Within days of Katrina's landfall, the national office coordinated a telethon with the BET channel and the American Red Cross to benefit victims.[65] The New Orleans affiliate, whose offices had been damaged during the hurricane, relocated to Baton Rouge and assisted victims while the staff themselves remained homeless. Nationwide, affiliates and the national office made hurricane response a high priority and assisted victims with food, shelter, and clothing. The organization's 2005 annual report stated that "By December 2005, our affiliates' tireless work had given over 30,000 Katrina survivors job training and employment, housing and counseling and placement services."[66] In fact, this approach to affiliate support by the national office was consistent with the League's five-year strategy, as reported in the group's annual report of its activities during 2005:

> The National Urban League's mission is to enable African Americans to secure economic self-reliance, parity, power and civil rights . . . To support our local affiliate leaders by assisting them in areas such as fundraising, financial management, marketing and governance. . . . Guided by this mission and strategy, the National Urban League is working and investing across the country to reduce economic disparities and help African Americans and others in need realize the American dream.[67]

Like the NAACP, the NUL responded to the devastation of Hurricane Katrina with a multilayered approach. The organization immediately issued calls for policy to aid victims and pressured Congress to make disaster relief its top priority:

> Congress [must] . . . immediately pass and fully fund comprehensive disaster assistance legislation that protects the right of victims of Hurricane Katrina . . . Congress' number one priority must be to help protect and restore the lives of the hundreds of thousands of citizens whose lives have been disrupted and destroyed.[68]

The Urban League specified the programs that Congress should implement, calling for a "Katrina Bill of Rights," which would include a Victims Compensation Fund, disaster unemployment assistance, and the protection of voting rights. The League considered these programs essential first steps that must be followed with additional congressional commitment to hurricane victims.[69] The "Katrina Bill of Rights" included calls for "the right of every neighborhood to return and rebuild . . . and the first right to work in rebuilding the Gulf Coast."[70]

Hurricane Katrina led the Urban League to reevaluate its priorities and to devote itself to addressing the inequities that the hurricane, and the government's response to the hurricane, revealed. In its 2005 annual report, the League noted the hurricane's impact on its future priorities and organizational focus:

> As 2005 ended, it seemed ironic that a hurricane had returned the Urban League Movement to its roots while defining its future. . . . In the future, the National Urban League will direct its energies to help close the economic gaps so vividly revealed by Hurricane Katrina with a renewed dedication and new strategy for the 21st century. . . . Hurricane Katrina underscored the critical need for this nation to focus its attention on the persistent issues of race, poverty, and the economic gap between Americans. Economic empowerment must be the civil rights agenda for the 21st century and the National Urban League Movement's programs, advocacy, and research will lead the way.[71]

As time passed after Katrina, the Urban League remained dissatisfied with the federal government's response to the crisis. In a speech at the St. Maria Gotti church in New Orleans in January 2006, Marc Morial, NUL president and CEO, called current rebuilding plans inadequate and made specific recommendations for improving the flood control and levee systems in New Orleans.[72] Explaining the League's ongoing relevance to the rebuilding and recovery efforts, Morial reported its service activities and advocacy in Congress and reiterated the call for a "Katrina Bill of Rights." Later that spring, he called on U.S. army secretary France J. Harvey "to establish an independent commission responsible for the immediate inspection of the nation's flood protection system."[73] Morial named the army's faulty response as the reason for such a commission:

> It is obvious that the U.S. Army Corps of Engineers has failed in its responsibility to protect urban Americans in hurricane-prone areas from Katrina-like disasters. That is exactly why an independent commission is needed to identify and rectify problems before it is too late.[74]

As plans were unveiled by the federal government, the state of Louisiana, and the city of New Orleans, the League was critical of proposals that it considered not beneficial to former residents. Upon the unveiling of the New Orleans Rebuilding Commission's plan for the return of hurricane victims, the Urban League issued a highly critical press release, claiming that the Commission's plans would prevent racially diverse neighborhoods from rebuilding:

> The New Orleans Rebuilding Commission's plan is exclusionary, disrespectful, and an affront to basic rights for any American citizen who wants to retain their own property and return to his/her own neighborhood ... Katrina survivors should be encouraged to return home; not turned away.[75]

Later in the spring of 2006, the League was critical of Homeland Security Secretary Michael Chertoff's plan to cut off housing vouchers for Katrina evacuees. "This [plan] is not only inhumane, but also shows the lack of competence and coordination in developing a comprehensive housing plan at both the local and national levels which the National Urban League called for in October 2005."[76]

In August 2006, the NUL issued a report called "Katrina: One Year Later." The report tracked the progress of proposals included in the "Katrina Bill of Rights" and highlighted League activities in support of hurricane survivors. It reiterated League calls for an independent commission to investigate what went wrong in the federal government's response to the hurricane, and for the redirection of various federal grants and funding toward hurricane recovery.[77] In addition to advocating the priorities of the Katrina Bill of Rights, as listed above, it reported that it had launched social service programs through thirty of its affiliates, particularly targeted at assisting hurricane survivors. The Report highlighted efforts to help survivors navigate the process to receive FEMA benefits, food, and shelter.[78]

Another area of League activity was its partnership with Freddie Mac, Citigroup, the Prudential Foundation, and the Citizens Charitable Foundation to establish the Katrina Fund. In August 2006, the League reported that $3.4 million had been raised by this fund to help the Gulf Coast region.[79] This type of business partnership made the League unique among civil rights groups, and the organization highlighted the success of the project through the press and in its annual report.

During its 2006 policy conference, the League focused attention on Congress and included the Katrina Bill of Rights as one of its four priorities. The organization also pressed both parties to commit to holding their 2008 national conventions in New Orleans, explaining that such a commitment would produce much needed income and demonstrate the country's overall support for rebuilding the city.[80]

The NUL's Ongoing Attention to Hurricane Katrina (2007–2008)

As Table 7.2 shows, the NUL continued its activities in support of Katrina survivors throughout 2007. The League was critical of the Bush administration, as well as Democrats in Congress, for their lack of attention to rebuilding New Orleans. Morial called for an action plan to reinvigorate recovery and rebuilding.

> I am making a call for the collective leadership on the federal, state and local levels to ensure the survival of one of our nation's greatest cities. Instead of finding fault and pointing fingers, I'd rather get our collective wits around the table to address this debacle before it becomes our nation's greatest shame.[81]

The League was dissatisfied and critical when President Bush failed to mention Hurricanes Katrina or Rita in his 2007 State of the Union address, and when the Democrats failed to mention the storms in their policy priorities for the first "100 hours" in Congress. "In the past year or so, there hadn't been a substantial additional piece of legislation passed related to fixing the utter devastation left in the wake of Katrina and Rita. There had been no provision, no funding to restore the levees and wetlands."[82] Morial expressed support for the Gulf Coast Hurricane Housing Recovery Act, which would provide $1.2 billion toward affordable housing in the region, but cautioned that chances at passage were slim because the legislation was tied to troop withdrawal from Iraq in the Senate, making it likely that President Bush would veto it. The League urged that the legislation be passed, and that the U.S. Senate not hold the plan "hostage by a debate over the Iraq War."[83]

On the second anniversary of the Hurricane, the League issued a public statement reiterating its own activities in Katrina's immediate aftermath and emphasizing its ongoing work:

> Since disaster first struck, the League hasn't let up in its efforts to get Katrina survivors back on their feet. In 2007, the National Urban League called for a National Katrina Summit, lobbied for swift passage of the Gulf Coast Hurricane Housing Recovery Act and teamed up with BP to launch the Gulf Coast Economic Empowerment to connect minority contractors with rebuilding work.[84]

The Gulf Coast Hurricane Housing Recovery Act emphasized the Katrina Bill of Rights' goal of "the right to return," and was therefore strongly supported by the League. The organization also spoke out concerning the mental health struggles of Hurricane survivors, linking the federal government's nonexistent housing policies to heightened anxiety among survivors.[85]

As mentioned above, the League also partnered with British Petroleum (BP) to develop the Gulf Coast Economic Empowerment Program (GCEEP), which targeted small and minority-owned construction firms in the Gulf Coast. As one component of the GCEEP, the NUL conducted a series of "Empowerment Tours," which put small and minority-owned firms in touch with contractors looking for assistance. It conducted multiple tours throughout the Gulf Coast in 2008 in locations such as Lake Charles, Louisiana, and Port Arthur, Texas.[86]

After Hurricane Gustav hit New Orleans in September 2008, the League issued careful, but limited, praise of the government's response. However, Morial's public statements pointed to the ongoing weakness of the levees, and urged the Army Corps of Engineers to quicken its work to strengthen the levees and protect wetlands:

> The Army Corps of Engineers has secured about $15 billion for a comprehensive repair and upgrade of the New Orleans region flood control system. I believe that is a necessary investment . . . I urge the Army Corps to step up the pace of its work. We must raise the height of the levees as well as strengthen them as quickly as possible. We must also be mindful of nature's own hurricane protection system and work to rapidly restore our nation's wetlands.[87]

Conclusion

The NUL and NAACP responses to proposals for welfare reform and to the crisis set off by Hurricane Katrina further demonstrate the importance, in the formulation of their priorities, of the interaction of conditions both internal and external to the organizations. During the welfare reform battles of the 1990s, the NAACP limited its responses because it was undergoing internal financial and organizational crises. The NUL was more aggressive because it considered welfare reform to be an important component of its newly defined mission, which was partially driven by its need to highlight its uniqueness as compared to the NAACP.

After their immediate responses to Hurricane Katrina, both the NUL and the NAACP gave less attention to the aftermath of the catastrophe. Both organizations shifted their attention to other issues because of an external condition—decreasing *national* attention to the hurricane. As the League explained, it considered itself to be a leader among civil rights organizations in their responses to Katrina and called its Katrina Bill of Rights a "clarion call" for other civil rights groups.[88] While the NUL saw Katrina as an opportunity to highlight its ongoing focus on economic inequities, the NAACP provided immediate responses without a larger commitment to making poverty issues a priority. As national attention faded, the NAACP decreased the attention paid to Katrina in the activity of its central office as well as in its guidance to its affiliates. On the other hand, the League's conception of itself as a leader in this area led the group to maintain its attention to anti-poverty policy on the national platform as well as in collaboration with local organizations.

Chapter 8

Conclusions

Because people wouldn't work for such low amounts of money, they were accused of being lazy—dependent on the government. In a real sense taking a job could put you further in poverty because you wouldn't qualify for aid. People didn't like living on public assistance. You know, they wanted to do something. An able-bodied man couldn't get a job, so he had to abandon the family to be sure that they were able to survive. . . . These policies were antithetical to building family, to strengthening family. Then they turn around and accuse the family.
   —Bernard Lafayette, founding member of SNCC, former SCLC National Program Administrator, National Coordinator of the 1968 Poor People's Campaign, interview with author, July 10, 2008

During the 1960s, local groups and affiliates of national civil rights organizations worked in African American communities throughout the South, and in northern cities, registering people to vote. Local workers for national organizations were consistently struck by the levels of poverty in these communities, and understood that one's economic concerns interacted with one's potential for political participation, making the latter less likely. Driven by these concerns, local organizations, and national staff working at the local level, pushed for a focus on economic equity by the civil rights movement.[1]

   After Congress passed Johnson's War on Poverty, many local organizations saw the program as an opportunity to have their anti-poverty efforts funded by the federal government. Once these local groups, including chapters of the NAACP, NUL, SNCC, and CORE, became involved with implementation of the War on Poverty, anti-poverty issues entered the national civil rights agenda. National offices, which had not recognized the growing importance of local anti-poverty efforts to the movement, were now behind the curve. The struggle to regain preeminence and relevance to the movement led national organizations, such as the NAACP and CORE, to prioritize anti-poverty policy. For the NUL and SNCC, groups that had been more consistently concerned with poverty issues, the War on Poverty was an opportunity to influence the civil rights agenda, and to solidify their positions within the civil rights issue niche. By the late 1960s, organizational competition within the civil rights issue niche had almost disappeared. The NAACP and NUL were concerned with maintaining themselves financially as other groups became inactive and disintegrated. These concerns, coupled with changes in the political environment, led both organizations to step away from advocacy for national, high-cost anti-poverty programs. In more recent history, both advocated on behalf of the poor when there was national attention devoted to the issue. Driven by their need to maintain their relevance, both groups sought to provide assistance to and advocacy on behalf of Katrina survivors.

In this chapter, I return to the questions posed at the beginning of this project. How do interest groups choose their priorities? When do the poor gain representation? As I note in Chapter 7, organizational archives are not yet available concerning the welfare reform battle of the 1990s or the response to Hurricane Katrina. Therefore, when addressing the reasons groups represent low-income African Americans, I rely on my analysis of the 1960s and 1970s. My findings indicate that organizational decision-making cannot be understood by examining either internal or external factors in isolation. Because of differences in each organization's structure, the NAACP, NUL, CORE, SNCC, and SCLC responded differently to organizational competition within their issue niche in their determination of priorities during the 1960s. By the early 1970s, changes in the external political environment drove the NAACP and NUL to reassess their attention to anti-poverty policy. Each organization's financial status, tactics, and structure determined how it responded to changes in the external environment.

Organizational decisions to represent the poor were sometimes strategic, sometimes based on an ideological commitment to represent the poor, and sometimes both. However, decisions were never purely ideological. Groups were always aware of strategy, and of their position within their issue niche, when determining their priorities. Even for SNCC, arguably the most ideologically driven group studied in this project, advocacy on behalf of the poor happened in part because of the group's acknowledgment of its effect on other civil rights organizations' priorities. Ideology is certainly relevant to group strategy—SNCC's rejection of the War on Poverty was driven by its own vision of economic justice. However, the findings in this project point to the importance of moving beyond ideology as an explanation for group priorities—a group has multiple ideological commitments; structural and strategic considerations will determine which commitments become organizational priorities.[2]

After returning to these questions that are central to the project, I discuss questions raised by this research that remain unanswered. For example, are these findings applicable to other issue niches and time periods? I present preliminary arguments that, in fact, these findings do apply to other groups of organizations in their decisions to advocate on behalf of subpopulations of their constituencies. This research also raises further questions about the factors that lead organizations to increase their advocacy on behalf of the poor. My findings indicate that organizations varied in their attention to anti-poverty policy. What explains this variation? What factors determine the *level* of attention a group devotes to anti-poverty policy? Finally, I discuss the implications of my findings on understandings of African American politics, and the representation of multiple interests within identity-based groups.

How Do Interest Groups Choose Their Priorities?

The organizations I examine in this project were consistently concerned with maintaining their memberships, or constituencies, and with maintaining themselves as organizations. Even for SNCC, which started off as a group opposed to any self-maintenance, concerns about survival led leadership to build an organizational bureaucracy. Groups chose priorities based on a sometimes very loose understanding of the goals that would please the people they claimed to represent. These findings are not particularly surprising, and support scholars' existing understanding of the influence of membership on organizational priorities (Wilson 1995 [1973]; Clark and Wilson 1961; Moe 1980). However, understanding that membership preferences matter to organizations does not tell us very much about how organizations choose the issues, or interests, they will represent. An organization's membership, or constituency, is broadly defined and will include multiple sets of interests. My findings shed light on how organizations determine the sets of interests they will represent, and why they arrive at these decisions.

Table 8.1 provides a summary of the findings in this project, and explains the interaction of internal and external factors for each instance of priority shift. Overall, my findings indicate that an organiza-

Table 8.1. Summary Table of Priority Shifts Explained in This Project

Period of shift	Organization	Direction of shift*	Expectations confirmed	Determinants of priorities explained
Early to mid-1960s (War on Poverty)	NAACP	Increase	• Centralized structure leads to concern with external local groups • Activities of rival organization expand NAACP priorities • Elites not particularly influential	• Competition drove NAACP to increase its advocacy on behalf of the poor; • NAACP structure allowed shift to occur and be successful at national and local levels
	NUL	Increase	• Changes to affiliate structure make anti-poverty grants priority for national office • National office seeks to preserve unique position within issue niche • Government funding possibility leads to restructuring	• Increasing national oversight of affiliates led NUL to receive War on Poverty grants. • NUL position within issue niche led it to restructure and pursue the grants
	SNCC	Increase	• Decentralized structure leads support for local anti-poverty programming, not War on Poverty. • National office considers itself "radicalizer" of other groups • Support of political elites for War on Poverty contributes to form of strong opposition to program	• SNCC commitment to local organizing led it to oppose War on Poverty and focus on local organizing • SNCC perception of its radicalizing role within the movement led it to vocally oppose War on Poverty and advocate for local solutions
	CORE	Increase	• Decentralized structure leads to little power by national office • National office feels internal competition from affiliates. Elites not particularly influential	• Growth led national office to be increasingly concerned with maintaining relevance to local offices • Despite reservations, national office increased attention to War on Poverty because local offices already active

Table 8.1. (Continued)

Period of shift	Organization	Direction of shift*	Expectations confirmed	Determinants of priorities explained
Mid- to late 1960s	CORE	Increase	• Changing national/affiliate structure leads national office to oversee local activities • Competition not particularly influential • Elites not particularly influential	• Because of its increasingly important role in CORE, national office oversaw local efforts to preserve War on Poverty funding.
	SCLC	Increase	• Changing national/affiliate structure leads national office to increase concern with local activities • Competition not particularly influential • Elites not particularly influential.	• Urban uprisings and exposure to northern poverty convinced SCLC staff that poverty was next phase of civil rights movement • SCLC reorganization and growth during mid-1960s allowed national campaign
Late 1960s to early 1970s	NAACP	Decrease	• External organizations facing decline; national organization no longer concerned with priorities of these groups • Competition less influential as organization regains preeminence. • Elites not particularly influential	• Organizational competition for membership, or potential membership, no longer existed for NAACP • Organization faced period of financial difficulty; returned to traditional priorities and strategies
	NUL	Decrease	• Changing national/affiliate structure leads to singular focus on local affiliate activities • Competition not particularly influential • Potential elite support leads to grassroots focus.	• External political changes made local organizing attractive for NUL, which sought federal funding. • Exclusive focus on local organizing precluded national focus on poverty.

*Increase: organization increases its advocacy on behalf of the poor; decrease: organization decreases its advocacy on behalf of the poor; as defined in Chapters 2 and 3.

tion's structure contributes to the priorities it chooses to pursue, but also how it implements those priorities. As I discussed in previous chapters, I expected that national organizational priorities would be influenced by local groups. My findings indicate that an organization's relationship with local offices consistently determined how it implemented its priorities, and sometimes the level of attention it gave to anti-poverty policy. These findings apply to multiple organizations with varying relationships with their local offices, such as SNCC and the NAACP. Although in-depth analysis of the 1990s and the response to Katrina is not possible, a cursory assessment of factors leading to organizational choices to represent the poor point to the importance of affiliate activities for both the NAACP and NUL—particularly in their immediate responses to Hurricane Katrina, when both groups were most active.

My findings are strengthened because the relationship between the national and local offices remained important to organizational decision-making even as groups underwent substantial structural changes. For example, during the War on Poverty, the NUL national office was committed to national-level advocacy on behalf of the poor. Affiliates were active, and the national office was engaged in programming of affiliates, but national-level advocacy was considered a primary function of the national office. During the late 1960s, on the other hand, the national office began to primarily focus on local-level organizing of and services for low-income African Americans. The national office considered one of its primary responsibilities to oversee, and direct, the programming of the affiliates. This change led the national office to step away from national-level advocacy and instead focus on local organizing. During each period, the national office's relationship with its local affiliates contributed to its level of advocacy on behalf of the poor. The national office's increasingly directive relationship with its affiliates during the mid-1960s allowed the organization to make the War on Poverty a national priority, and to receive substantial EOA grants. The group's shift in focus to local organizing during the late 1960s and early 1970s led the NUL to step away from national-level advocacy.

As Table 8.1 summarizes, my findings indicate that each organization considered its position within the issue niche as it determined its priorities during the 1960s. For some groups, such the NAACP and SNCC, this position was particularly important for determining the group's goals. During the mid-1960s, each group's priorities were affected by the relations among groups within the civil rights issue niche. By the late 1960s and early 1970s, competition was less influential on group priorities. As my expectations predicted, because rival organizations were no longer determining the important issues for the entire issue niche, organizations such as the NAACP and NUL determined their priorities without concern about the activities of other groups—a contrast to their substantial concerns during the 1960s.

My findings also support the argument that an organization's relationship with political elites will affect its goals, although primarily when organizations are receiving government funding. As McAdam (1982) argues, the influence of elites will vary based on the tactics and goals of the organization. The NUL was quite concerned with attracting and maintaining the support of political elites—it received government funding to conduct its programming throughout the 1960s and early 1970s. SNCC was also concerned with the support of political elites, but from a very different perspective than the NUL. SNCC was vocally, and adamantly, opposed to the Johnson administration during the War on Poverty. As discussed in Chapter 5, this opposition was based on SNCC's ideological opposition to federal aid programs, but also because it maintained SNCC's role as a "radicalizer" of other groups. SNCC needed to retain its distance from mainstream policymakers; staff and supporters considered this distance to be critical to SNCC's purpose. Although my findings support those of existing scholarship that point to the influence of specific internal and external factors on decision-making, my research indicates that examining either type of factor in isolation does not allow for a complete understanding of the influences on organizational priorities. Both internal structural factors and external factors, such as competition and elite support, are critical to understanding why organizations shift their priorities.

While this project is unique within the interest group literature because it examines priority shifts among multiple organizations during multiple legislative periods, these findings should be further tested by examining organizations in other issue niches, and during other time periods. Additionally, this research contributes to an understanding of when groups, which are marginalized within an organization's constituency, gain political representation. Drawing on the work of Cohen (1999) and Strolovitch (2007), this research begins an examination of the factors that lead to such representation. Organizations must have particular incentives to represent politically vulnerable groups among their constituencies. Additionally, groups will remain within their general "identity," even when offering such representation. Although antipoverty policy, and the political language surrounding welfare reform, was largely framed as a critique of African American women beginning in the late 1960s, civil rights organizations did not shape their responses with much attention to gender. Instead, and with a few exceptions, organizations addressed poverty issues with little attention to the intersection of race, gender, and class inherent in policy reform. Even as they shifted their priorities, civil rights organizations framed their attention to class-based policy within their existing focus on racial equality generally—they did not amend this focus to include an approach that recognizes the variety of oppressive experiences among their constituencies.

This research opens the door for further understanding of whether interactions between structural and external variables, such as organizational competition, determine whether other groups represent the interests of politically marginalized subgroups of their constituencies. Future research may examine the effect of interorganizational competition on gay and lesbian groups' decisions to include transgendered rights in their mission statements beginning in the mid- to late 1990s. Prior to the 1990s, mainstream organizations argued that transgender issues should be separate from gay and lesbian rights issues; for example, a national employment nondiscrimination law need not protect transgendered individuals.[3] Once local transgendered rights groups increased their political activism and began to work with local gay rights groups, national organizations found it in their best interest to include transgendered interests in their mission statements, and to lobby on behalf of inclusion of transgendered individuals in a national nondiscrimination law.[4]

Future research might also examine how low-income immigrant groups fare in the larger immigrant rights movement, how lesbian rights became incorporated into the women's movement of the 1970s, or how civil rights organizations began to address crime and drug issues during the late 1980s and 1990s. Analysis of these cases will provide further understanding of how interest groups choose the issues they will represent, and how politically marginalized groups gain representation. The findings in this project point to the importance of external factors, such as competition among organizations, but also to paying particular attention to structural differences among groups within the same issue niche, and the effect of these differences on the interests a group chooses to represent.

How Do the Poor Gain Representation? Findings and Future Research

My analysis demonstrates that national organizations, which consider economic equity to be a secondary priority, advocate on behalf of the poor when they have incentives to do so. For mainstream groups, these incentives may come in the form of government funding or membership retention. Because of competition from local organizations, national groups may find it necessary to shift their priorities to the interests of marginalized groups. More radical organizations play a pivotal role in increasing representation in the U.S. political system because they compete with more conservative organizations for their constituencies—not because their representation affects long-term policy change or is particularly effective in representing the interests of marginalized groups. Based on the research in this project, it is the organizations that selectively, and strategically, choose to represent the poor that survived. Groups that prioritize the representation of the poor from their inception have a much more difficult time maintaining themselves. Future research outside the civil rights issue niche would contribute to existing literature on the viability of organizations founded to represent the poor, and the possibilities for increasing their longevity.[5]

In this project, I assessed organizations' advocacy on behalf of the poor without any discussion of the effectiveness of such representation. To facilitate analysis of decision making across organizations and time periods, I limited my focus to national-level activities concerning welfare reform, with the exception of my discussion of Hurricane Katrina. This approach allowed me to compare organizational activities pertaining to pieces of legislation that are commonly understood to affect the poor. Future research might draw distinctions among the types of representation each organization provided for the poor, and the factors that led to each type. It is not particularly surprising that SNCC focused on grassroots mobilization to establish local anti-poverty programs, or that the NAACP focused on lobbying strategies. Which strategies were more effective in representing the interests of the poor? Can representation be considered effective if it does not involve mobilization of the people an organization claims to represent?

My research in this project establishes and explains shifts in priorities within organizations. However, civil rights organizations varied in their level of attention to the poor, and in the magnitude of their shifts in priorities (see Figure 5.1). The NAACP and CORE experienced the most substantial shift during the War on Poverty. SNCC and the NUL advocated on behalf of the poor during the early 1960s, making their shifts less dramatic. CORE and the SCLC increased their attention substantially during the late 1960s, while the NUL maintained the same high level of attention to anti-poverty policy it had committed during the War on Poverty. During the early 1970s, both the NAACP and NUL decreased their attention to approximately half of what it had been during the late 1960s. The NAACP and NUL also decreased attention to welfare policy after TANF reform passed—after Katrina, the NAACP dropped its level of attention more substantially than the NUL (see Figure 7.1). What explains the differences in the magnitudes of the shifts in priority among civil rights organizations?[6]

A brief consideration of the groups might indicate that the differences could be explained by an organization's ongoing concern with the needs of the poor—SNCC and the NUL, two organizations with a founding commitment to poverty issues, experienced the least dramatic increase in attention during the War on Poverty. The research in this project demonstrates that differences in founding ideologies do not explain these differences. The SCLC was also committed to advocacy on behalf of the poor, but did not choose to address anti-poverty legislation until the late 1960s. Future research is necessary to explore the factors that lead to differences in the levels of attention organizations devote to anti-poverty issues.

Throughout the post-civil rights era, civil rights groups' representation of the poor has fluctuated among, and within, the organizations. Although each group rhetorically supported economic equity, and considered issues such as employment discrimination to be critical to the civil rights struggle, few gave consistent priority to anti-poverty issues.[7] The findings in this project point to the problems with assuming common priorities or interests within identity-based groups. Practically, it is not surprising that organizations must decide on a hierarchy of goals; however, it is important to note that civil rights organizations did not choose to represent low-income African Americans solely because of a broadly defined commitment to racial equality—high levels of identification and concern with issues of black poverty do not necessarily translate into advocacy by largely middle-class organizations.[8]

Representing the poor is a taxing endeavor, both financially and organizationally. For organizations not embedded in a community, leaders must establish relationships and trust with community leaders before any mobilization can occur, and often before national representation can be effective.[9] Other goals, which are less expensive and have a higher possibility for success, are more attractive for interest groups to pursue, pointing to a well-documented aspect of American democracy: it is difficult for the interests of the poor to be heard in Congress, by political parties, or by interest groups.[10] Although they may be more inclined to share political and economic concerns with low-income African Americans, civil rights organizations face the same disincentives to such representation as other interest groups.[11] Despite these challenges to the representation of the poor, the findings in this project offer a glimmer of hope for increasing the representation of marginalized interests within the U.S. political system. If one organization in a movement can be convinced of the interests of a politically alienated group, other organizations may follow suit, and representation may become increasingly democratic.

Appendix A

Archival Research and Coding

> Anyone passing by the files . . . could easily get the impression that this
> organization runs on paper. It is certainly true that the maintenance of records is
> vital to the conduct of our business . . . But, there has to be a limit somewhere
> . . . I urge that before sending anything to the files, you ask yourself whether it is
> really necessary to do so. . . . When in doubt, throw it out.[1]
> —Dr. John Morsell, Assistant Director, NAACP,
>   to Executive Staff, April 4, 1962

I found the document quoted above as I sat in a dark microfilm room
researching the NAACP files. Needless to say, it was disconcerting. When
in doubt, throw it out? Realistically, of course, organizations cannot
keep all the paper they generate. In the case of the NAACP during the
1960s, I was reassured by the remainder of the memo cited above, which
pleaded with employees not to keep *copies* of memos and documents.
Such a document points to the benefits and problems with archival
research. Examining organizational files allows a researcher to gain a
sense of an organization and its operations. The researcher is not
required to base his or her conclusions on surveys of staff, who may or
may not have accurate memories of meetings, activities, or the workings
of the organization outside of their department. On the other hand,
conclusions based on this research rest solely on the researcher's interpretation of documents and events. In addition to trusting the analysis,
the reader must rely on the researcher to accurately report on the state
of archives. In this appendix, I first present information on the archives

of each organization: their location, size, and completeness. Second, I present my research process: my decision about which documents to consult, how I coded them, and how I analyzed them. In addition to archival research, I interviewed former and current leadership and staff. In the final section of this appendix, I provide details about the interview process and questions asked.

The Location and State of the Archives

The research for this project is based on the organizational archives of the Congress of Racial Equality, National Association for the Advancement of Colored People, National Urban League, Southern Christian Leadership Conference, and Student Nonviolent Coordinating Committee. When I began my research on this topic, I found that many of the organizations' archives had been microfilmed, and that Northwestern University's library owned the microfilmed collections. I traveled to the archives of two organizations housed at the Library of Congress. The archives made my task of researching five organizations doable. It also gave me confidence in my future findings. If I was attempting to understand the internal dynamics that led to priority change, I needed to be able to analyze as complete a collection of internal documents as possible.

The archives of each organization are composed of their office files. Some include both national and branch offices, and others include only the national office. Generally, I restricted my research to the national office files of each organization. If, however, a branch's files were relevant to a particular anti-poverty campaign, or to a national decision to reach out to branches, I consulted those files.

Not surprisingly, each organization varied in its record-keeping. An organization's approach to record keeping may reflect its approach to bureaucracy. For example, the NAACP and NUL files are more extensive than those of the SCLC and SNCC. However, both SNCC and the SCLC maintained national office files and records. Although relying on archives for extensive documentation of the fieldwork for either group would be difficult, the national offices did function bureaucratically. In the following sections, I describe the size and state of each organization's archives. To give an additional sense of the differences among the amount of materials in each organization's archives, I provide the length of time I spent examining each group's documents.[2]

CORE Archives

CORE's organizational archives have been microfilmed in two sets: *The Papers of the Congress of Racial Equality 1941–1967* and an *Addendum* that includes material between 1944 and 1968. The material in the *Addendum* was not released to the public until after the publication of the *Papers* collection. The *Papers* collection is housed at the State Historical Society of Wisconsin. The *Addendum* collection is housed at the Martin Luther King, Jr. Center for Nonviolent Social Change in Atlanta. The *Papers* collection is 49 microfilm reels of over 60,000 pages of files. The *Addendum* collection includes 25 reels.[3]

The bulk of the files in the *Papers* collection spans the period between 1959 and 1964. They include six series, with National Director's files and files of each department.[4] The bulk of the files in the *Addendum* collection spans the period between 1961 and 1969. The *Addendum* includes seven subgroups, with National Director's files, Community Relations Department files, and Organization Department files. Both microfilmed collections are organized as the original files from the national office were when they were delivered to the MLK Center and the Historical Society.[5]

The *Papers* collection includes all the files that were delivered to the Historical Society. The *Addendum* collection excludes some employment and project applications. Excluded documents are noted in the guide to the collection—the index for each subgroup lists any files that were not microfilmed.[6]

I spent two days tracking down the guides to the microfilmed collections—the Northwestern University Library held the microfilm, but the guides were lost. After finding the guides at the Carter G. Woodson Regional Library in Chicago, I spent about two weeks examining the microfilmed collections.

NAACP Archives

The NAACP archives are housed at the Library of Congress, Manuscript Division. Parts of the microfilmed collection run through the early 1970s. I examined materials from the late 1950s through the late 1960s on microfilm. I examined printed material from the late 1960s through the early 1970s at the Library of Congress. To examine material less than 25 years old at the Library of Congress, a researcher must have written permission from the NAACP.[7]

The microfilmed archives of the NAACP are enormous, and continue to grow as documents become publicly available. In fact, during the course of this project, additional material, which I examined at the Library of Congress, has become available on microfilm. The collection currently includes 1,292 reels of microfilm. It is divided into thirty parts and their supplements. Of course, much of the collection documents the NAACP earlier history and is not relevant to my project. I examined the following Parts of the NAACP collection:

1. Supplement to Part 1, Meetings of the Board of Directors, Records of Annual Conferences, Major Speeches, and Special Reports[8]
2. Supplement to Part 4, Voting Rights, General Office Files
3. Supplement to Part 10, Peonage, Labor, and the New Deal
4. Supplement to Part 13, NAACP and Labor
5. Supplement to Part 16, Board of Directors Files
6. Supplement to Part 17, National Staff Files
7. Part 21, NAACP Relations with the Modern Civil Rights Movement
8. Part 29, Branch Department Files

Each Part includes numerous series and subgroups and is filmed on numerous reels. For example, the Supplements to Part 1 and 16 each include 12 reels; Part 29 includes 18 reels.

The microfilmed NAACP papers are edited by John H. Bracey and August Meier, two well-established scholars of the history of civil rights organizations. Each Part of the collection is indexed, and each index includes a statement of any files that were not microfilmed. For example, in the guide to the supplement to Part 17, the editors note that "One subseries of the staff materials was not selected for edition: Applications for Positions."[9]

The NAACP files at the Library of Congress are also organized by parts. I visited the Library to examine the archives from the 1970s. I examined materials in the following parts:

1. Part IV: Office File[10]
2. Part VII: Gilbert Jonas Co.[11]
3. Part VIII: Administrative File[12]
4. Part IX: Washington Bureau[13]

Similar to the microfilmed collection, each of these Parts includes numerous series and subgroups. The Office and Administrative files include files from the boards of directors; annual convention files are housed in the Administrative collection; the Washington Bureau collection houses all of the office's administrative documents and legislative reports. The collections vary in size: the Washington Bureau collection is held in 569 containers; the Administrative file is held in almost 500 containers; the Gilbert Jonas Co. collection, the records of the NAACP's relationship with its PR firm, is smaller and is held in approximately 108 containers.[14]

I spent about two months examining the microfilmed collections of the NAACP. I visited the University of Chicago library to examine national staff files and to the Roosevelt University library to examine a full collection of *The Crisis*. I made two trips to the Manuscript Division at the Library of Congress, and spent approximately two weeks in sum examining the files from the 1970s. I also visited the Library of Congress Reading Room to examine the NAACP's annual reports.

NUL Archives

The NUL archives are not available on microfilm, and are housed at the Library of Congress, Manuscript Division. Similar to the NAACP, permission from the League is required to access materials less than twenty-five years old. I examined the files of the Office of Washington Operations and the national office. The national office files include approximately 166,600 items and are housed in approximately 430 containers.[15] The Office of Washington Operations files include approximately 26,100 items and are housed in approximately 50 containers.[16] I spent two weeks at the Library of Congress examining the League's archives.

SNCC Archives

The SNCC Archives are housed at the State Historical Society of Wisconsin. They are available on microfilm in their entirety, and are recorded on 73 reels. Most of the papers cover the period between 1960 and 1968, the height of SNCC activities.[17] The collection is divided into three subgroups: the Atlanta (National) Office, the New York Office, and the Washington Office. I examined materials in each of the three subgroups.

The microfilmed collection is organized into the same folder and subgroup headings as the collection at the King Center. As the editors point out in the guide, often the logic of the organization of the materials is difficult to discern. Files are not organized consistently—some documents are filed chronologically, while others are not. As the Guide editors state: "The researcher. . . . must be flexible in approaching the SNCC papers, and must realize that the occasional apparent lack of order reflects a great deal about SNCC's operations as an organization."[18]

The SNCC archives are rich, and include lengthy transcripts of meetings among national staff (not minutes of meetings, but verbatim transcripts). Because such documents take longer to examine than letters or meeting minutes, which are often categorized by topic, I spent approximately four weeks examining the SNCC archives.

SCLC Archives

The SCLC Archives are available at the Dr. Martin Luther King, Jr. Center for Nonviolent Social Change in Atlanta, Georgia. The microfilm collection is divided into four parts: Records of the President's Office, Records of the Executive Director and Treasurer, Records of the Public Relations Department, and Records of the Program Department. The collection is filmed on 72 reels. John H. Bracey, Jr., and August Meier are the general editors of the microfilm collection.

The index of each part lists any records that were not filmed. The records of the president's office are complete except for tape recordings; the records of the executive director and treasurer are complete except for some treasury reports; the Public Relations Department Records are complete except for a series of "routine financial records"; and the records of the Program Department have been filmed in their entirety, with the exception of artifacts, such as denim jackets worn during the Poor People's Campaign.[19]

The SCLC archives were the first I examined. I was still forming my criteria for which documents to examine, and therefore I looked at many more than for other organizations. I spent approximately four weeks on this task.

Collecting and Analyzing Archival Materials

Step One: Consulting Indexes of Archives and Pulling Documents

I approached each organization's index with a list of my topics of interest. Generally, I looked for index subjects that pertained to organizational priorities, decision making, structure, poverty efforts, relations between policymakers and organizations, relations between national and local offices, and relations among organizations. I would then note each document listed under a subject, and examine those documents. Of course, the index subjects in each organization's archive varied. For example, I examined documents pertaining to NUL New Thrust Initiative; no other civil rights organization had a New Thrust Initiative entry in its index. Table A.1 is a list of the terms searched in the SCLC's archive. Although this list is specific to SCLC, it demonstrates the types of entries I examined in each organization's archives.

Table A.1. SCLC Subject Index Items Searched

1962 Amendments to the Social Security Act	Fundraising techniques
Account balances	Guaranteed income
Affiliates	Guaranteed income proposal
Annual conventions—planning, program, resolutions, reports	Individual and community development
Annual reports	Job creation programs
Antipoverty legislation	Legislative task force
Antipoverty programs	Major issues
Anti-welfare laws	Mass action
Budget	Mass meetings
Citizen's Crusade Against Poverty	Messages of support
Community antipoverty workers	Minimum wage
Community questionnaire	Mississippi Freedom Democratic Party
Congress, U.S. antipoverty legislation	NAACP
Contributions	NUL
CORE	Nixon, Richard M.
Crusade for Opportunity	OEO
Democratic National Committee	Operation Breadbasket
Democratic Party	Operation Breadbasket
Department of Affiliates	Poor People's Campaign
Department of Economic Affairs	Poverty
Direct action	Poverty bill
Direct action programs	President's reports
Direct action projects	Questionnaire relating to SCLC
Donations	Republican National Committee
Economic system, U.S.	Republican Party
Employment, guaranteed	Requests for information
EOA Amendments	SCLC summer project
EOA of 1964	SNCC
Executive board	SNCC-SCLC contributions
Executive board meetings	Social Security Act
Executive committee	Spring Mobilization in Washington
Field reports	Surveys, SCLC
Finance office	Teacher surveys
Financial office report	Washington Bureau
Financial reports	Welfare reform
Full Opportunity Act of 1967	Welfare rights organization
Fundraising	Work programs

I searched for materials based on their subject; however, the collections are generally not organized by subject. Once I formed a list of documents I planned to examine, I created a spreadsheet of the reel numbers, or box numbers, and the documents on each reel or in each box. I then sorted the spreadsheet by reel or box number, allowing me to examine multiple documents of interest that might be housed on the same reel or in the same box. I then either requested containers from a

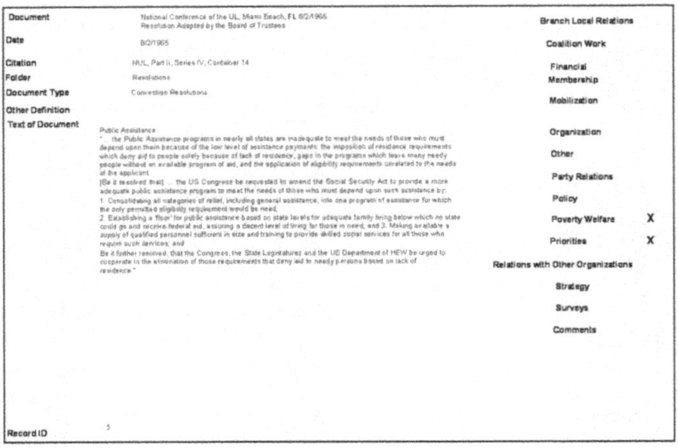

Document: National Conference of the UL, Miami Beach, FL 8/2/1965
Resolution Adopted by the Board of Trustees

Date: 8/2/1965

Citation: NUL, Part II, Series IV, Container 14

Folder: Resolutions

Document Type: Convention Resolutions

Other Definition

Text of Document: Public Assistance
"... the Public Assistance programs in nearly all states are inadequate to meet the needs of those who must depend upon them because of the low level of assistance payments, the imposition of residence requirements which deny aid to people solely because of lack of residence, gaps in the programs which leave many needy people without an available program of aid, and the application of eligibility requirements unrelated to the needs of the applicant.
[Be it resolved that] ... the US Congress be requested to amend the Social Security Act to provide a more adequate public assistance program to meet the needs of those who must depend upon such assistance by:
1. Consolidating all categories of relief, including general assistance, into one program of assistance for which the only permitted eligibility requirement would be need,
2. Establishing a 'floor' for public assistance based on state levels for adequate family living below which no state could go and receive federal aid, assuring a decent level of living for those in need, and 3. Making available a supply of qualified personnel sufficient in size and training to provide skilled social services for all those who require such services; and
Be it further resolved, that the Congress, the State Legislatures and the US Department of HEW be urged to cooperate in the elimination of those requirements that deny aid to needy persons based on lack of residence."

Record ID: 5

Branch Local Relations
Coalition Work
Financial
Membership
Mobilization
Organization
Other
Party Relations
Policy
Poverty Welfare X
Priorities X
Relations with Other Organizations
Strategy
Surveys
Comments

Figure A.1. Example of data entry template.

librarian in the Manuscript Reading Room, or examined documents on the microfilm machine. In both cases, I photocopied any document of interest. After researching the five organizations, I had approximately six file boxes of photocopied archival material.

Step Two: Coding Documents

After collecting an organization's materials from microfilm or the Library of Congress, I began the second phase of my research process: coding the archival documents. I did not start researching another organization's archives until all the material from the previous organization had been coded. First, I filed the documents in folders based on their content, and sometimes their type. Similar to the searched index terms, the name of folders were consistent across organizations, with few exceptions. Each organization has folders titled "Annual Reports," "Financial Records," "Structural Concerns," and "Staff Concerns." But, only the SCLC has a folder titled "Poor People's Campaign." After filing, I entered each organization's materials into a database. Each organization has its own database, although I used the same template for each one. Using the same template provided consistency in the coding process, and facilitated comparisons among organizations.

Figure A.1 is an example of an entry from the NUL files during the 1960s.[20] The fields on the left reflect information about the document.[21] The "Document Type" field is a drop-down menu of possible choices,

Table A.2. Number of Documents Collected

Organization	Documents collected/database entries
CORE	439
NAACP 1960s	335
NAACP 1970s*†	217
NUL 1960s*∞	203
NUL 1970s*	105
SCLC	295
SNCC	281

*Materials collected at Library of Congress. The photocopying process in the Manuscript Reading Room is more expensive and labor-intensive than copying at a microfilm machine. By the time I visited the Library of Congress, I had researched four organizations on microfilm. I had a defined sense of what types of documents I was looking for, and what types were not relevant to my project. Therefore databases based on Library research include fewer documents than those researched on microfilm.
†Includes data relevant to discussion of NAACP post-War on Poverty activities from 1966 and 1967.
∞Includes extensive data relevant to discussion of NUL activities concerning a guaranteed income and the Family Assistance Plan in 1968 and 1969.

such as "message to membership," "external message," and "internal communication." The "Text of Document" field is unrestricted in terms of the amount of information that can be entered. I entered relevant quotes, and sometimes summarized the documents, into this field.

The fields on the right reflect the type of "evidence" the document provides. Each field is a drop-down menu with two choices: a blank, or an X. As Figure A.1 illustrates, multiple fields may be selected. I often make notes in the "Comments" field about the significance of a particular quote in the document; or, when there are multiple "evidence" categories checked, the relevance of quotes to the checked categories.

The process of coding the archival materials was lengthy, and sometimes took longer than collecting the documents. Generally, I allocated three weeks to coding the materials from each organization's archives. The size of each database varies, and reflects the number of documents I collected from each organization. Table A.2 lists the number of entries in each database.[22]

Step Three: Analyzing the Documents

After I entered the documents into each organization's database, I exported the evidence fields to a spreadsheet, and sorted documents by the type of evidence they provided. I then sorted those documents by topic and chronologically. For example, I separated all of the documents pertaining to an organization's priorities. I then organized these documents based on whether they were evidence of an internal discussion of priorities or public documents reflecting an organization's priority, such as a convention program.

Once I sorted the documents, I wrote extensive analyses of the evidence in each category. These write-ups were part of the research process; each organization's write-up for a time period was over 100 pages. The write-ups allowed me to have a complete story of the priorities of the organization at the time, and to assess the various factors influencing priorities. The case study of each organization was based on its write-up.

Interviews with Leadership and Staff

After completing archival research on each organization, I attempted to track down and interview former leadership and staff. Additionally, I interviewed more recent leaders and staff about organizational responses to the 1990s welfare reform legislation and Hurricane Katrina. Overall, I sent twenty former and current leaders and staff requests for interviews. Two of the people I contacted were infirm, and I heard from their caregivers that they would be unable to be interviewed. I interviewed three former leaders: Dr. Bernard Lafayette, the former coordinator of the SCLC Poor People's Campaign; John Lewis, former chair of SNCC; and Hugh B. Price, former president and CEO of NUL. I talked to two current leaders, Avis Jones-DeWeever, the director of research, public policy, and information at the National Council for Negro Women; and a second civil rights leader who wished to remain anonymous. I engaged in an e-mail exchange with Julian Bond, chair of the board of the NAACP, and former SNCC leader.

Although my questions during each interview varied based on the organization's former and current activities, all interviews were constructed around two overall areas: the organization's attention to poverty and the organization's decision-making process. I adjusted the following questions to be relevant to each leader's experience:

1. Was your organization concerned with economic issues?
2. What form did this concern take? Direct action within communities? Legislative lobbying at the national level? State level?
3. What type of economic issues was your organization concerned with? Issues like social security and unemployment? Or anti-poverty policy?
4. What was your organization's reaction to the [relevant anti-

poverty legislation]? Did you think that the [relevant anti-poverty legislation] could be successful?

5. Did your organization consider [relevant anti-poverty legislation] to be important to its mission?

In addition to questions pertaining to an organization's approach to antipoverty, I also asked questions concerning organizational decision making:

1. How did your organization determine what its priorities would be?
2. Did your board of directors focus on big-picture directives, or was it involved with day-to-day decision-making?
3. Did the national staff decide the organization's main focus, and then tell local organizations? Or did local organizations influence national priorities?

Because these were open-ended, semistructured interviews, many questions emerged during them. For example, my interview with Dr. Lafayette focused on the Poor People's Campaign, its purpose, organizing challenges, and victories of the campaign.

I interviewed Lewis and Jones-DeWeever in Washington, D.C.; Lafayette in Kingston, Rhode Island; and Price in New Rochelle, New York. All interviews lasted between forty-five and ninety minutes. They were recorded and then transcribed.

Magnitude of Shifts in Organizational Attention to Anti-Poverty Policy

In addition to understanding *when* and *why* organizations shifted their attention to anti-poverty policy, it may also be important to consider differences among organizations in the *level* of attention devoted to such policy. The following tables demonstrate that decisions to advocate on behalf of the poor were a bigger departure from ongoing anti-poverty activities for some organizations than for others.

Table B.1. Organizational Attention to Anti-Poverty, Early and Mid-1960s

Organization	Level of attention, early 1960s	Level of attention, War on Poverty	% point change	Magnitude of change
NAACP	8%	57%	49	+ 6.13
CORE	5%	27%	22	+ 4.40
SNCC	22%	41%	19	+ 0.86
NUL	59%	100%	41	+ 0.69
SCLC	16%	8%	− 08	− 0.50

Shift analyzed in Chapter 5. Author's calculations, as presented in Chapter 3.

Table B.2. Organizational Attention to Anti-Poverty, Mid- and Late 1960s

Organization	Level of attention, mid-1960s	Level of attention, late 1960s	% point change	Magnitude of change
SCLC	8%	73%	65	+8.12
CORE	27%	68%	41	+1.51
NUL	100%	100%	0	+0.00
SNCC	41%	19%	−22	−0.54
NAACP	57%	38%	−19	−0.33

Shift analyzed in Chapter 5. Author's calculations, as presented in Chapter 3.

Table B.3. Organizational Attention to Anti-Poverty, Late 1960s and Early 1970s

Organization	Level of attention, late 1960s	Level of attention, early 1970s	% point change	Magnitude of change
NUL	100%	56%	−44	−0.44
NAACP	38%	19%	−19	−0.50

Shift analyzed in Chapter 6. Author's calculations, as presented in Chapter 4.

Table B.4. Organizational Attention to Anti-Poverty Between 1995–1996 and 1997–1998

Organization	Level of attention, 1995–1996s	Level of attention, 1997–1998	% point change	Magnitude of change
NUL	40%	24%	−16	−0.40
NAACP	17%	10%	−7	−0.41

Shift calculated in Chapter 7. Author's calculations, as presented in Chapter 7.

Table B.5. Organizational Attention to Anti-Poverty Between 2005–2006 and 2007–2008

Organization	Level of attention, 1995–1996	Level of attention, 1997–1998	% point change	Magnitude of change
NUL	70%	59%	−11	−0.16
NAACP	49%	22%	−27	−0.55

Shift calculated in Chapter 7. Author's calculations, as presented in Chapter 7.

Abbreviations

ADC	Aid to Dependent Children
AFDC	Aid to Families with Dependent Children
CCAP	Citizens' Crusade Against Poverty
CAP	Community Action Program
CORE	Congress of Racial Equality
EOA	Economic Opportunity Act
FAP	Family Assistance Plan
FOR	Christian Fellowship for Reconciliation
HEW	Department of Health, Education, and Welfare
NAACP	National Association for the Advancement of Colored People
NLUCAN	National League on Urban Conditions Among Negroes
NUL	National Urban League
NWRO	National Welfare Rights Organization
PPC	Poor People's Campaign
OEO	Office of Economic Opportunity
SCLC	Southern Christian Leadership Conference
SNCC	Student Nonviolent Coordinating Committee
TANF	Temporary Aid to Needy Families

Chapter 1. Anti-Poverty as a Civil Rights Issue?

1. Polling in the immediate aftermath of Katrina exposed different perceptions of the Bush administration's response for African Americans and whites. A Pew Research Center poll revealed that 83 percent of African Americans and 63 percent of whites believed President Bush had not moved quickly enough with relief efforts. See Frymer, Strolovitch, and Warren 2006.

2. Barbara Bush, *Marketplace* radio program, National Public Radio, September 5, 2005.

3. On the racial implications of welfare policy, the equation of African Americans with welfare recipients, and the negative implications of this association see, for example, Gilens 1999; Omi and Winant 1994; Lieberman 1998; Quadagno 1994.

4. See Jackson 2007; Hamilton and Hamilton 1997; Carson 1995.

5. John Lewis, interview with author, June 11, 2008.

6. See Appendix A for detailed information about archival holdings and analysis. The archives of the NAACP, SNCC, SCLC, and CORE are available in their entirety on microfilm through the late 1960s. NUL archives are housed at the Library of Congress, Manuscript Division, Washington, D.C. NAACP archives are also housed in their entirety at the Library of Congress, Manuscript Division. For materials during the 1960s, I relied on the collection as microfilmed: John H. Bracey, Jr., and August Meier, *Papers of the NAACP* (1995a–f). For materials beginning in the late 1960s, I relied on the archives at the Library of Congress. SNCC archives, housed at the Martin Luther King, Jr. Center for Nonviolent Social Change in Atlanta, are available on microfilm, *The Student Nonviolent Coordinating Committee Papers, 1959–1972* (New York: New York Times Company Microfilming, 1982). CORE archives are housed at two locations: the State Historical Society of Wisconsin and the Martin Luther King, Jr. Center for Nonviolent Social Change. CORE papers are available on microfilm, *The Papers of the Congress of Racial Equality, 1941–1967* (Sanford, N.C.: Microfilming Corporation of America, 1988) and *The Papers of the Congress of Racial Equality, Addendum: 1944–1968* (Ann Arbor, Mich.: University Microfilms International, 1982). SCLC archives are available, with the exception of the Treasurer's Department,

on microfilm from the *Black Studies Research Sources*. Materials from the Treasurer's Department are incomplete, and are available at the King Center (Bracey and Meier, 1995g).

7. Extensive research examines the internal structure of groups and the influence of structure on group operations. I am more specifically interested in the influence of internal structural factors on priority-setting and decision-making. Works that focus on internal dynamics and their influence on priority-setting include Moe 1980; Rothenberg 1992; McFarland 1984; Barakso 2004. On the internal structures of organizations and the significance of structure to group operations, without specific application to priority-setting, see, for example, Michels 1949; Lipset, Trow, and Coleman 1956; Truman 1960 [1951]; Greenstone 1969; Hrebenar and Scott 1982; Bacharach and Lawler 1982; J. Wilson 1995 [1973]; Clemens 1997; Polleta 2004.

8. See Barakso 2005; Tierney 1994; and Baumgartner and Leech 1998.

9. See Lowi 1979; Gamson 1975; Ross 1970; Heinz, Laumann, Nelson, and Salisbury 1993; Baumgartner and Leech 2001; Berry 1999; Walker 1991.

10. See Goluboff 2007 on the NAACP's shift away from labor issues after *Brown v. Board of Education*. See Frymer 2008 on NAACP attention to labor issues, and explanations of institutional constraints faced by the organization when addressing such issues. See Hamilton and Hamilton 1997 on civil rights organizations' attention to economic policy generally.

11. NAACP involvement with some unions such as the AFL-CIO, which was part of the implementation of the War on Poverty, could have increased the organization's attention to Johnson's antipoverty policies. The NAACP labor department recognized the large number of potential NAACP members in the trade union movement (on Labor Department engagement with unions, see Frymer 2008). Although attention to the preferences of union members on policy may have contributed to the NAACP position on, and public statements about, the War on Poverty, it did not require that the War on Poverty become a top priority for the organization. Concern with addressing the needs of members, however, certainly included cross-membership with unions. See Chap. 5 for more detailed discussion of NAACP concern with membership retention in the determination of its priorities.

12. Public support for welfare declined dramatically beginning in the early 1960s. In response to the question, "Are we spending too much, too little, or about the right about on welfare?" the proportion of Americans supporting increased welfare spending dropped from 60 percent in 1961 to just below 40 percent in 1969 and to 20 percent in 1973. The proportion of Americans stating that too much is spent on welfare increased from just less than 10 percent in 1961 to just less than 30 percent in 1969, and to over 50 percent in 1973 (Teles 1996, 44). See Teles (1996) for a detailed discussion of the reasons for shifting public support for AFDC policy. Also see Lieberman 1998; Gilens 1999; Quadagno 1994.

13. By the late 1960s, the NAACP had become less dependent on membership for revenue because of its increasing reliance on grants from the Ford and Rockefeller Foundations and the Carnegie Corporation; see Marger 1984, 26. Marger explains that NAACP foundation funding was unique among civil rights organizations because it received nonspecific grants. Other organizations, such as CORE and SCLC, received foundation funding, but for specific projects.

14. Histories of civil rights organizations refer to shifts in focus to poverty issues, but their purpose is not to trace the organization's commitment to social

welfare policies; therefore, such shifts are examined only when they involved an overall change in the organization's focus (see Peake 1987; Kellogg 1967; Garrow 1986; Meier and Rudwick 1973; Carson 1995; Parris and Brooks 1971). Exceptions include Jackson 2007, discussed above. Another exception is an article by Meier and Bracey, in which they analyze the history of the NAACP from its founding to 1965 in terms of its adherence to the ideals of the progressive movement, and the influences of environmental and internal factors on the organization's programs and strategies (Meier and Bracey 1993, 4). The authors claim that internal struggles did not influence the direction of the organization, and that the NAACP remained flexible in its prioritization of issues. Based on environmental changes, the organization was able to incorporate economic issues without moving away from its initial focus on racial policies (20). Like Hamilton and Hamilton 1997, Meier and Bracey's 1993 analysis of economic issues does not include public assistance policies.

15. See Mink 1998; Giddings 1984; Hancock 2004.

16. See Giddings 1984; Ransby 2003.

17. On Aid to Families with Dependent Children rates, see Piven and Cloward 1993 [1971], 194; on discrimination against eligible African Americans, see Lieberman 1998.

18. For ideology as an explanation for organizational behavior, see Jackson 2007.

19. See Appendix A for detailed discussion of interviews.

20. For example, Rothenberg's analysis of Common Cause's decision to shift priorities to a focus on the MX missile assesses only the internal factors that led to the shift, and is limited to decision-making within one organization and concerning one issue (Rothenberg 1992). Similarly, Barakso's (2004) analysis of decision-making in NOW is intentionally limited to analyses of internal dynamics and structural influences.

21. See Baumgartner and Leech 1998; Walker 1991; Hrebenar and Scott 1982; Gray and Lowery 1996; Browne 1998; Berry 2003; Salisbury 1984; Tarrow 199; McFarland 1992.

22. For an example of this type of analysis, see Browne 1998.

23. On the importance of internal structures, particularly the role of membership to organizational priorities, see Barakso 2004, 2005.

24. NAACP, "NAACP: Its History, Policy, Program, Structure, and Staff," June 23, 1957, Group 3, Series A, Reel 7.

25. *New York Times,* January 28, 1912, 11, as cited in Morris 1984, 49.

26. Membership in a Community Chest was not easy to achieve. The affiliate had to qualify as an independent social service agency, according to a city's philanthropic board (Moore 1981, 57).

27. "Core Statement of Purpose," January 1960, Series VI, Publications, No. 26, Reel 49, Frame 468.

28. See "What Is CORE," January 1960, Series VI, Publications, No. 26, Reel 49, Frame 462.

29. Ella Baker as cited in Giddings 1984, 384. Ella Baker, interview, Civil Rights Documentation Project (Moorland-Springarn Collection, Howard University, Washington, D.C.), 34–35.

30. Constitution and By-Laws of SCLC, Part 2, Subgroup 2, 1957, Reel 1.

31. Ibid.

32. SNCC, "Statement of Purpose, April 1960 Founding Conference," Subgroup A: Atlanta Office, 1959–1972, Series 1: Chairman's Files 1960–1969, April 16, 1960, Reel 1.

33. SNCC, "Report of the Fall Conference of the Student Non-Violent Movement," Subgroup A: Atlanta Office, 1959–1972, Series V: SNCC Conferences, Section 4: October 14–16, October 17, 1960, Reel 11, Frame 433.

34. SNCC, "Letter Concerning October Conferences and Recommendations of the Temporary SNCC, October 14–16, 1960," Subgroup A: Atlanta Office, 1959–1972, Series 1: Chairman's Files 1960–1969, October 17, 1960, Reel 1.

Chapter 2. Assessing and Explaining Shifts in Organizational Priorities

Epigraph: NAACP, Part IX, Box 26, Memo to the Presidents and Secretaries of Branches, Youth Councils and College Chapters, From: the Executive Director, September 28, 1966; emphasis original.

1. See Appendix A for a detailed discussion of each organization's archives and my method of selecting and coding documents in the archives.

2. The activities assigned to these categories are based on surveys of interest group activities in the legislative arena, as well as social movements. On interest group activities, see Heinz et al. 1993; McFarland 1984; Goldstein 1999; Scholzman and Tierney 1986; Walker 1991; Moe 1980. On social movement organization activities, see Zald and McCarthy 1987; McAdam 1982; Chong 1991; Morris 1984.

3. NUL, Report on Recommendations and Resolutions Passed by the 1964 Delegate Assembly, August 1, 1964, Part II: The Records of the National Urban League, 1960–1966, Series VI, Box 21 .

4. NAACP, Board of Directors Meeting Minutes, September 14, 1964, Supplement to Part I, 1960–1965, Group 3, Series A, Box A26, Reel 1.

5. Additionally, based on archival research, I cannot be sure that I am capturing *all* reports of *all* activities. Instead, archives allow me to report, as thoroughly as possible, the variety of types of activities in which groups engaged. Secondary reports, such as stories in newspapers, would provide the opportunity to gauge the total number of organizational activities. However, I am measuring activities that were not counted by secondary sources. For a count of sit-ins as reported by the *New York Times*, for example, see McAdam 1982.

6. NAACP, Memo to Presidents of Branches and State Conferences from Roy Wilkins, Re: Action Memo: NAACP in the War on Poverty, October 13, 1964, Supplement to Part 17, National Staff Files, 1956–1965, Group 3, Series A, Box A-310.

7. Moe 1980 explains that subgroups have difficulty gaining influence in the larger organization if the subgroup is not resource rich. Without the influence subgroups gain by pooling their resources, the larger organization has little incentive to pay attention to their interests (91). Often, the subgroups that form with interests in advocating on behalf of the poor are not the poor themselves, but rather middle-class individuals who are ideologically committed to helping the poor. Therefore, they will not be as committed to withholding their resources from the larger organization on behalf of the poor.

8. Rothenberg's findings pertain to Common Cause, a public interest organization offering purposive and expressive benefits to its members. On the particular ideological and political commitment of members of civil rights organizations, see Wilson 1995 [1973] and Bayes 1992.

9. See Haines 1988 for a discussion of the "radical flank effects" on civil rights organizations. See Tarrow 1994 on the importance of face-to-face interac-

tions within social movements and the impact of cycles of protest and the inter-action among elites, which may lead to reform.

10. Scholars have found, however, that organizations that rely on large donors are less likely to mobilize low-income individuals than are organizations that plan protests and boycotts (Kollman 1998; Goldstein 1999).

11. Scholars have found that an organization has particular incentive to maintain relations with its membership when other groups with similar missions share the group's constituency (McFarland 1984, 106; Berry 1984, 95; Clark and Wilson 1961, 157–61; Wilson 1995 [1973], 266).

12. See Clark and Wilson 1961; Wilson 1995 [1973]; Schattschneider 1960; Lowi, 1969; Heclo 1978; Heinz et al. 1993; Baumgartner and Leech 2001; Gray and Lowery 1996.

13. In response to the pluralist understanding of high levels of competition among groups, scholars argue access to the political system is limited to certain groups representing powerful interests. (Schattschneider 1960; McConnell 1966; Lowi 1969; Ross 1970; Cater 1964). In fact, competition among groups is quite low because organizations carve out areas of interest, and strive to main-tain autonomy within that area (Heinz et al. 1993; Browne 1998).

14. Other examples of citizen groups sharing constituencies include lesbian, gay, bisexual, and transgendered (LGBT) groups and women's organizations. Also, more issue-based groups, such as environmental groups, might consider themselves to represent the interests of a defined constituency—environ-mentalists.

15. NAACP, letter to Miss L. Pearl, Board Member, from Gloster B. Current, June 14, 1961, Supplement to Part 16, Board of Directors Files, 1956–1965, Group 3, Series A, Box 27.

16. Whitney Young, NUL executive director, testified before the House Com-mittee on Education and Labor concerning the EOA in 1964. He also testified before the Senate Committee on Finance concerning the FAP in 1970. Clarence Mitchell, director of the NAACP Washington Bureau, testified before the Senate Committee on Finance on alternatives to the FAP in 1972. Hearing appearances based on the *CIS/Index to Publications of the U.S. Congress*. I examined the list of witnesses and their affiliations for each hearing conducted in the House and Senate on the 1964 EOA and the 1972 FAP.

Chapter 3. Civil Rights Organizations and the War on Poverty

Epigraph: Whitney Young, "A Cry from the Dispossessed," *Christian Century*, December 14, 1964, NUL, Part II: The Records of the National Urban League 1960–1966, Series V, Box 35.

1. Congressional Quarterly Service 1965, 1255–56.

2. On advocacy efforts leading up to the War on Poverty, see Noble 1997; Quadagno 1992; Flanagan 2001; Hays 2001; Patterson 1994. On organizing and activism during the implementation of the War on Poverty, see, for example, Naples 1998.

3. See Giddings 1984.

4. See Abramovitz 2000; Hancock 2004; Giddings 1984.

5. See Bond et al. 2009; Jonas 2005.

6. NAACP, NAACP Annual Convention Resolutions 1961, Supplement to Part I, 1960–1965, Group 3, Series A, Box A13.

7. See Abramovitz 2000; Giddings 1984.

8. NAACP Annual Convention Resolutions 1962, Supplement to Part I, 1960–1965, Group 3, Series A, Box A-14.

9. NAACP, "The Convention Speaks to Staff," August 1, 1962, Supplement to Part I, 1960–1965, Group 3, Series A, Box A-12.

10. NAACP, Report of the Secretary to the Board of Directors for the Month of January 1964, February 10, 1964, Supplement to Part I, 1960–1965, Group 3, Series A, Box A-32.

11. NAACP, Board of Directors Meeting Minutes, September 14, 1964, Supplement to Part I, 1960–1965, Group 3, Series A, Box A-26.

12. NAACP, Executive Committee Meeting Minutes, October 13, 1964, Supplement to Part I, 1960–1965, Group 3, Series A, Box A-26.

13. NAACP, Report of the Secretary to the Board of Directors for the Month of September 1964, October 13, 1964, supplement to part I, 1960–1965, Group 3, Series A, Box A-32.

14. NAACP, "NAACP Maps Plans for Anti-Poverty Program," *The Crisis* 71, 9 (November 1964): 616.

15. NAACP, Report of the Secretary to the Board of Directors for the month of October 1964, November 9, 1964, Supplement to Part I, 1960–1965, Group 3, Series A, Box A-32.

16. NAACP, NAACP Annual Convention Resolutions 1965, Supplement to Part I, 1960–1965, Group 3, Series A, Box A-20.

17. NAACP, Memo to Roy Wilkins from Herbert Hill, Re: Federal anti-poverty program, January 11, 1965, Supplement to Part 17, National Staff Files, 1956–1965, Group 3, Series A, Box A-310.

18. NAACP, Board of Directors Meeting Minutes, April 12, 1965, Supplement to Part I, 1960–1965, Group 3, Series A, Box A-26.

19. NAACP 1966, 19.

20. See Dickerson 1998; Hamilton and Hamilton 1997.

21. NUL, "Resolution Adopted by the Delegate Assembly at the 1963 National Conference of the Urban League, Los Angeles," August 1, 1963, Part II, Series IV, Box 14.

22. NUL, Memo to: National Agencies, American Leaders, Local Urban Leagues, From: National Urban League, Re: The Current Attack on ADC in Louisiana, September 19, 1960, Part II: The Records of the National Urban League, 1960–1966, Series II, Box 1.

23. NUL, Memo to: Executive Secretaries of Affiliated Organizations, From: Lester B. Granger, January 18, 1961, Part II: The Records of the National Urban League, 1960–1966, Series II, Box 1.

24. NUL, Memo to: Executive Secretaries, Local Urban Leagues, From: Nelson C. Jackson, Associate Director, Re: ADC Activities and specifically the State of Louisiana matter, February 6, 1961, Part II: The Records of the National Urban League, 1960–1966, Series IV, Box 13. The national office included this explanation before any testimony in front of legislative committees, and encouraged affiliates to do the same. See Memo to: Local Executives, NUL Professional Staff, From: Whitney Young, January 1964, Part II: The Records of the National Urban League, 1960–1966, Series I, Box 27.

25. NUL, Letter to Myles B. Amend, Chairman, State Board of Welfare, New York, From: Henry Steeger, July 6, 1961, Part II: The Records of the National Urban League, 1960–1966, Series I, Box 47.

26. Ibid.

27. NUL, "Public Welfare Problems and Trends as Expressed by Urban

League Affiliates," May 1, 1962, Part II: The Records of the National Urban League, 1960–1966, Series IV, Box 16.

28. NUL, Memo to: Urban League Staff; From: Jeweldean Jones, Associate Director, Health and Welfare, Re: Pending Health and Welfare Legislation, May 14, 1962, Part II: The Records of the National Urban League, 1960–1966, Series IV, Box 14.

29. NUL, Letter to Mr. I. Jack Fasteau, Chief, Special Standards Group, Division of Welfare Services, Department of Health, Education, and Welfare, June 20, 1963, Part II: The Records of the National Urban League, 1960–1966, Series IV, Box 13.

30. NUL, Resolution Adopted by the Delegate Assembly at the 1963 National Conference of the Urban League, Los Angeles, August 1, 1963, Part II: The Records of the National Urban League, 1960–1966, Series IV, Box 14.

31. NUL, Press Release: "Urban League Official Cites 'Panic Button' Distortion of Welfare as Grave Danger to Social Work 'Balance," December 6, 1963, Part III: The Records of the National Urban League, 1967–1979, Box 45.

32. NUL, Letter to President Johnson from Young, January 15, 1964, Part II: The Records of the National Urban League, 1960–1966, Series I, Box 19.

33. NUL, Press Release, April 9, 1964, Part II: The Records of the National Urban League, 1960–1966, Series I, Box 27.

34. The NUL is not a membership-based organization. Therefore, a lack of membership mobilization does not indicate less priority to policy. In my quantification of priority levels, mobilization of membership is not applied to the NUL. I gauge the organization's financial commitment not through membership fund-raising but through attempts to receive corporate or foundation funding for its anti-poverty activities.

35. NUL, Summary and Recommendations: NUL War on Poverty Workshop, May 20, 1964, Part II: The Records of the National Urban League, 1960–1966, Series I, Box 38. .

36. NUL, Board Meeting Minutes, May 21, 1964, Part III: The Records of the National Urban League, 1967–1979, Box 170.

37. NUL, Summary and Recommendations: NUL War on Poverty Workshop, May 20, 1964. .

38. NUL, Memo to: Leo Bohanon, Raymond Brown, Clarence Coleman, Cernoria Johnson, Henry Talbert, From: Nelson C. Jackson, June 3, 1964, Part III: The Records of the National Urban League, 1967–1979, Box 75.

39. NUL, Letter to Shriver from Young, June 15, 1964, Part II: The Records of the National Urban League, 1960–1966, Series I, Box 19.

40. NUL, Summary Report of the 1964 National Conference, August 1964, Part II: The Records of the National Urban League, 1960–1966, Series VI, Box 21.

41. Ibid.

42. NUL, Memo to Leo Banano, Raymond Brown, Clarence Colement, Nelson Jackson, Henry Talbert, From: Cernoria D. Johnson, June 16, 1964, Part II: The Records of the National Urban League, 1960–1966, Series I, Box 19.

43. NUL, Resolutions and Recommendations adopted by delegate assembly at the 1964 National Conference of the Urban League, August 1, 1964, Part II: The Records of the National Urban League, 1960–1966, Series IV, Box 14.

44. NUL, Press Release announcing Community Action Assembly, October 3, 1964, Part II: The Records of the National Urban League, 1960–1966, Series V, Box 33.

45. NUL, Press Release, December 10, 1964, Part II: The Records of the National Urban League, 1960–1966, Series V, Box 5;, Remarks Before Community Action Assembly, Health and Welfare Session, Jeweldean Jones, December 10, 1964, Part II: The Records of the National Urban League, 1960–1966, Series V, Box 5;, Address by Anthony J. Celebrezze, Secretary of HEW, at the Community Action Assembly, December 10, 1964.

46. NUL, *NUL Annual Report 1964–1965*, 1966, Part III: The Records of the National Urban League, 1967–1979, Box 1667.

47. NUL, Press Release, "NUL Hold Poverty Workshops in the South," January 25, 1965, Part II: The Records of the National Urban League, 1960–1966, Series V, Box 35.

48. NUL, Memo to Whitney Young, From: Reginald Johnson, May 14, 1965, Part II: The Records of the National Urban League, 1960–1966, Series I, Box 28.

49. NUL, Memo to Young, From: Cernoria D. Johnson, Re: Report on NUL/OEO Relationships, February 2, 1965, Part II: The Records of the National Urban League, 1960–1966, Series I, Box 87.

50. NUL, Press Release: 1965 National Conference of the Urban League, August 5, 1965, part II: The Records of the National Urban League, 1960–1966, Series V, Box 35.

51. NUL, National Conference of the Urban League, Miami Beach, Resolution Adopted by the Board of Trustees, August 2, 1965, Part II: The Records of the National Urban League, 1960–1966, Series IV, Box 14.

52. Ibid.

53. CORE, as summarized in the 22nd Annual National Convention, National Director's Report, July 2, 1964, Addendum, Series C, National Action Council and Conventions, No. 80, Reel 9, Frame 786; Minutes of the 1962 CORE national convention, July 2, 1962, Series I: National Director's File, No. 23, Reel 2, Frame 557.

54. CORE, See "Statement on District Welfare Story," August 17, 1962, Series I, National Director's Files, No. 89, Reel 6, Frame 77; Letter from James M. Quigley, Assistant Secretary, HEW to James Farmer, March 20, 1962, Series V, Departments and Related Organizations, No. 168, Reel 28, Frame 36.

55. CORE, Memo to Steering Committee from Norman Hill, re: Summer Project—North, April 26, 1963, Series V, Departments and Related Organizations, No. 132, Reel 26, Frame 451.

56. CORE, Minutes of the 1963 CORE Convention, June 30, 1963, Series IV, National Action Council, No. I, Reel 16, Frame 500.

57. CORE, Memo to NAC, From: Normal Hill, Program Director, Re: Major Party Convention Project, Series IV: National Action Council, No. 3, Reel 16, Frame 706.

58. CORE, Statement from Norman Hill, National Program Director, June 29, 1964, Series V, Departments and Related Organizations, No. 123, Reel 25, Frame 711.

59. CORE, 22nd Annual National Convention, National Director's Report, July 2, 1964, Addendum, Series C, National Action Council and Conventions, No. 80, Reel 9, Frame 786.

60. CORE, Memo to Chapter Chairmen, From Department of Organization, January 27, 1965, Addendum, Subgroup B, Associate National Director's Files, no. 32, Reel 9, Frame 121.

61. CORE, See Memo to George Wiley from James T. McCain, Re: Job Speci-

fication and Recent Activities, January 25, 1965, Series V, Departments and Related Organizations, No. 293, Reel 38, Frame 935.

62. CORE, NAC Minutes, February 6–7, 1965, Series IV: National Action Council, No. 5, Reel 16, Frame 1037.

63. CORE in the Field, Bag IV, June 25, 1965, Addendum, Subgroup E, Community Relations Department, Series I, No. 24, Reel 10, Frame 438; CORE in the Field, October 1, 1965, Bag 69, Addendum, Subgroup E, Community Relations Department, Series I, No. 24, Reel 10, Frame 467; CORE in the Field, Bag 71, November 1, 1965, Addendum, Subgroup E, Community Relations Department, Series I, No. 24, Reel 10, Frame 469.

64. CORE in the Field, Bag 71, November 1, 1965, Addendum , subgroup E, Community Relations Department, No. 24, Reel 10, Frame 469.

65. CORE in the Field, Bag I, June 22, 1965, Addendum, Subgroup E, Community Relations Department, Series I, No. 24, Reel 10, Frame 469; CORE in the Field, Bag V, June 28, 1965, Addendum, Subgroup E, Community Relations Department, Series I, No. 24, Reel 10, Frame 439; CORE in the Field, Bag VI, July 8, 1965, Addendum, Subgroup E, Community Relations Department, Series I, No. 24, Reel 10, Frame 440; CORE in the Field, Bag IX, July 9, 1965, Addendum, Subgroup E, Community Relations Department, Series I, No. 24, Reel 10, Frame 442; CORE in the Field, Bag 47, September 7, 1965, Addendum, Subgroup E, Community Relations Department, No. 24, Reel 10, Frame 458; *CORE-lator*, March–April 1965, No. 11.

66. CORE, Memo from Professor Mike Miller, NYU, "CORE and the War on Poverty," October 19, 1965, Addendum, Subgroup A, National Directors' Files, James Farmer, No. 81, Reel 3, Frame 58.

67. CORE, Memo from Judith Nussbaum, Re: Proposed Plans for Summer 1965, April 1, 1965, Research/Federal Programs, Series V, Departments and Related Organizations, No. 132, Reel 26, Frame 477.

68. CORE, NAC Minutes, April 10–11, 1965, Series IV: National Action Council, No. 5, Reel 16, Frame 1039.

69. CORE, 1965 Convention Schedule, July 1, 1965, Series IV: National Action Council, No. 1, Reel 16, Frame 576.

70. CORE, Annual Report to the National CORE Convention by James Farmer, July 1, 1965, Addendum, Subgroup C, National Action Council and Conventions, No. 99, Reel 9, Frame 916.

71. CORE, Memo to CORE Chapter Chairman, From George Wiley, Associate National Director, November 10, 1965, Addendum, Subgroup B, Associate National Director's Files, No. 5, Reel 8, Frame 622.

72. CORE, Press Release: Poverty Program Cutback Assailed by CORE Official, November 8, 1965, Series V, Departments and Related Organizations, No. 193, Reel 31, Frame 186.

73. CORE, Press Release, April 3, 1966, Addendum, Subgroup E, Community Relations Department, Series III, Public Relations Files, No. 104, Reel 13, Frame 952; News Release, May 6, 1966, Subgroup E, Community Relations Department, Series III, Public Relations Files, No. 104, Reel 13, Frame 968.

74. CORE, *CORE-lator*, March 1, 1967, Addendum, Subgroup A, National Directors' Files, No. 24, Reel 5, Frame 335.

75. CORE, Press Release, May 24, 1966, Subgroup E, Community Relations Department, Series III, Public Relations Files, No. 104, Reel 13, Frame 978.

76. CORE, Press Release, September 26, 1966, Subgroup E, Community Relations Department, Series III, Public Relations Files, No. 104, Reel 13, Frame 1018.

77. CORE, NAC Meeting—December 31, 1965–January 2, 1966, January 2, 1966, Addendum, Subgroup C, National Action Council and Conventions, No. 1, Reel 107, Frame 992.

78. Ibid.

79. Despite McKissick's intentions, this formal retraining was never implemented. CORE, CORE's Policy of New Direction, February 1, 1966, Addendum, Subgroup A, National Directors' Files, Floyd McKissick, No. 28, Reel 5, Frame 399.

80. CORE, "A Nation Within a Nation," CORE's proposal for economic development and control of black areas (an economic New Deal for poor America), April 1, 1968, Addendum, Subgroup A, National Directors' Files, Floyd McKissick, No. 32, Reel 5, Frame 650.

81. SCLC, Part 1, Constituent letter to King from EK Evans, February 19, 1963, Reel 4.

82. SCLC, Part 1, Letter to Walter Reuther, 1964, Reel 4.

83. SCLC, Part 3, "Resolution of the Board, Annual Board Meeting, Southern Leadership Conference, April 13, 1966," 1966, Reel 9, Box 132.

84. SCLC, Part 3, "Resolution of the Board, Annual Board Meeting, Southern Leadership Conference, April 13, 1966," 1966, Reel 9, Box 132.

85. SCLC, Part 3, Memo to King from R. T. Blackwell, January 27, 1966, Reel 3, Box 45.

86. SCLC, Part 4, Statement by Dr. Martin Luther King, Jr., December 4, 1967, Reel 28, Box 179. Although the PPC became SCLC's movement, it was originally conceived by the National Welfare Rights Organization, a group of women welfare recipients. Although the SCLC eventually had to turn to the NWRO for its support of the PPC, the NWRO remained disheartened by the SCLC's command of the movement and lack of cooperation with this previously organized group of recipients (see Giddings 1984).

87. Dr. Bernard Lafayette, Interview with author, July 10, 2008, Kingston, Rhode Island.

88. SCLC, Part 3, Press Release: "Dr. King Touring Nation in Poor People's Campaign," March 17, 1968, Reel 5, Box 125.

89. SCLC, part 4, Internal memoranda, March 17, 1968, Reel 27, Box 179.

90. SCLC, Part 4, Memo from Albert Turner to Hosea Williams, Director of Mobilization, April 3, 1968, Reel 27, Box 177.

91. SCLC, Part 3, Form letter to affiliates, April 20, 1968, Reel 5, Box 125.

92. These pledges were never accompanied by policy changes that satisfied the PPC. SCLC, Part 4, "Poor People's Campaign Answer to the Response of Agency Meetings," June 12, 1968, Reel 27, Box 177.

93. SCLC, Part 4, Press Release, June 23, 1968, Reel 27, Box 178.

94. SCLC, Part 4, "Abernathy Speaks from Resurrection City," July 17, 1968, Reel 26, Box 177.

95. SNCC, Minutes of the SNCC Executive Committee Meeting, December 27–31, 1963, Subgroup A, Atlanta Office, 1959–1972, Series II: Executive and Central Committees, 1961–1967, Reel 3, Frame 329.

96. Ibid.

97. SNCC, "Some Comments on the Civil Rights Movement, reprinted from the *New York Herald Tribune*," May 23, 19, Subgroup A, Atlanta Office, 1959–1972, Series VII: Communications Department, 1960–1968, Reel 14, Frame 329.

98. SNCC, "Federal Programs—some notes and suggestions," March 29,

1965, Subgroup A, Atlanta Office, 1959–1972, Series VIII: Research Department, 1959–1969, Reel 21, Frame 1022. SNCC's critique of federal anti-poverty programs was consistent with the organization's ongoing critique of the federal government and of both political parties. For example, in his speech at the March on Washington, John Lewis pointed to the federal government's indictment of civil rights workers in Albany, Georgia, the inadequacies of both political parties for African Americans, and asked "Where is our party? Where is the political party that will make it unnecessary to have Marches on Washington?" As quoted in Carson 1995, 94.

99. SNCC, Minutes, Executive Committee, September 4, 1964, Subgroup A, Atlanta Office, 1959–1972, Series II: Executive and Central Committees, 1961–1967, Reel 3, Frame 353.

100. SNCC, Minutes at Waveland Retreat, November 1964, Subgroup A, Atlanta Office, 1959–1972, Series V: SNCC Conferences, 1960–1964, Reel 11, Frame 958.

101. SNCC, Life with Lyndon in the Great Society, vol. 1, no. 1, January 22, 1965, Subgroup A, Atlanta Office, 1959–1972, Series VII: Communications Department, 1960–1968, Reel 21, Frame 353.

102. Ibid., 1, no. 6, March 4, 1965.

103. Ibid., 1, no. 41, November 11, 1965, 3.

104. Ibid., 1, no. 13, May 1, 1965.

105. Ibid., 1, no. 44, December 2, 1965.

106. SNCC, Press Release: Poorest Counties Get Least Help, August 4, 1965, Subgroup A, Atlanta Office, 1959–1972, Series VII: Communications Department, 1960–1968, Reel 14, Frame 439.

107. Ibid.

108. SNCC, Fundraising Letter re: Poor People's Corporation, April 1, 1965, Subgroup A, Atlanta Office, 1959–1972, Series XVII: Other Organizations, 1959–1969, Reel 44, Frame 280.

109. SNCC, Minutes of the First Membership Meeting of the Poor People's Corporation, August 29, 1, Subgroup A, Atlanta Office, 1959–1972, Series VII: Communications Department, 1960–1968, Reel 44, Frame 280.

110. SNCC, A paper answering a few questions some people have raised in regards to the Poor People's Corporation, June 15, Subgroup A, Atlanta Office, 1959–1972, Series VII: Communications Department, 1960–1968, Reel 44, Frame 280.

111. SNCC, Minutes of Central Committee meeting, October 22–23, 1966, Subgroup A, Atlanta Office, 1959–1972, Series II: Executive and Central Committees, 1961–1967, Reel 3, Frame 608.

112. SNCC, "Position on Freedom Budget—CONFIDENTIAL—NOT TO BE LEAKED TO THE NEW YORK TIMES—NOT FOR PUBLIC CONSUMPTION," November 22, 1966, Subgroup A: Atlanta Office, 1959–1972, Series IV: Executive Secretary Files, 1959–1972, Reel 11, Frame 327.

113. SNCC, "Don't Shut Me Out! Some Thoughts on How to Move a Group of People from One Point to Another or Some Basic Steps Toward Becoming a Good Political Organizer," February 1, 1967, Subgroup A, Atlanta Office, 1959–1972, Series I: Chairman's Files, 1960–1969, Reel 2, Frame 1317.

114. SNCC, Report from Chairman, May 5, 1967, Subgroup A, Atlanta Office, 1959–1972, Series III: Staff Meetings, 1960–1968, Reel 3, Frame 1135.

Chapter 4. Civil Rights Organizations' Anti-Poverty Activities
During the Late 1960s and Early 1970s

Epigraph: NAACP, Statement of Clarence Mitchell, Director of the Washington Bureau and Legislative Chairman of the LCCR before the House Committee on Education and Labor on OEO Legislation, March 31, 1971, Part IX, Box 169.

1. See Hays 2001 for an analysis of groups engaged in advocacy concerning the FAP.

2. On the advocacy push for, and response to, the FAP see Hays 2001; Nadasen 2005; Quadagno 1994; Naples 1998.

3. NAACP, "CORE: The National Publication of the Congress of Racial Equality, October 1971, Convention Issue—Change and Growth," October 1, 1971, Part VIII: 1965–1999, Box 155, emphasis in original.

4. New York to Director, FBI, "SNCC," May 10, 1971, as cited in Carson, 298.

5. See Bond et al. 2009; Jonas 2005.

6. NAACP, Letter to Clarence Mitchell, Director, Washington Bureau NAACP from Gloster B. Current, Director of Branches and Administration, Re: Letter from Aaron Henry to Robert Weaver, March 7, 1966, Part IV: National Office, 1965–1975, Box A32.

7. NAACP, Memo to: NAACP branch presidents and Economic Opportunity, Church, Labor and Industry, Youth work and Community Coordination Committee Chairmen, August 4, 1966, Part IV: National Office, 1965–1975, Box A90.

8. NAACP, Memo to Roy Wilkins and John A. Morsell from Gloster B. Current, November 27, 1967, Part IV: National Office, 1965–1975, Box A19.

9. NAACP, Memo to: NAACP branch presidents . . . , August 4, 1966.

10. NAACP, Memo to Mr. Roy Wilkins, From: Richard W. McClain, Administratively Confidential, July 26, Part IV: National Office, 1965–1975, Box 90.

11. Ibid., emphasis in original.

12. NAACP, Memo to Wilkins; Thru: Richard McCalin, Robert Saunders, Virna Canson, From: Maurice Dawkins, Subject: A Policy for NAACP member participation in non-profit neighborhood economic development corporation, July, Part IV: National Office, 1965–1975, Box 90.

13. NAACP: 59th Annual Convention Resolutions, June 24–29, 1968, Part IV: National Office, 1965–1975, Box A7.

14. Ibid.

15. NAACP, Statement of Clarence Mitchell, Director, Washington Bureau, NAACP, before the House Committee on Ways and Means on HR 14173, October 23, 1969, Part IX, Washington Bureau, Box 169.

16. NAACP, Convention Resolutions 1970, July 11, 1970, Part VIII: 1965–1999, Box 1.

17. NAACP, *Annual Report*, 1971.

18. NAACP, Roy Wilkins column about Welfare Reform Bill, July 7, 1971, Part IX: Washington Bureau, Box 140.

19. *New York Times*, September 9, 1971, 19.

20. NAACP, 63rd Annual Convention Resolutions, July 3–7, 1972, Part VIII: 1965–1999, NAACP.

21. NAACP, *Annual Report*, 1972.

22. NAACP, *Annual Report*, 1973.

23. NAACP, Letter to Ms. Doris L. Lynch from Clarence Mitchell and NAACP national office in NY, November 22, 1972, Part IX: Washington Bureau, Box 140.

24. NUL, Program Planning for Health and Welfare, Annual Convention, September 1966, Part II: The Records of the National Urban League, 1960–1966, Series IV, Box 14.

25. NUL, Resolutions Adopted by the NUL Delegate Assembly at the 1966 Conference of the Urban League, August 3, 1966, Part III: The Records of the National Urban League, 1967–1979, Box 211.

26. NUL, Press Release, December 21, 1966, Part III: The Records of the National Urban League, 1967–1979, Box 287.

27. NUL, Memo #1, To: All Urban League Executives, From: SAV-CAP Committee, December 16, 1966, Part III: The Records of the National Urban League, 1967–1979, Box 287.

28. NUL, *Washington Bureau Newsletter,* 1, no. 4, June 30, 1967, Part III: The Records of the National Urban League, 1967–1979, Box 287.

29. NUL, Testimony of William J. Haskins, Associate Director, National Urban League, Washington Bureau before the President's Committee on Civil Disorders, October 7, 1967, Part III: The Records of the National Urban League, 1967–1979, Box 56.

30. NUL, "A New Thrust for the Urban League Movement," June 5, 1968, Part III: The Records of the National Urban League, 1967–1979, Box 35.

31. Ibid.

32. NUL, "Building Ghetto Power," Speeches presented at the 58th Annual NUL Conference, New Orleans, July 28–August 1, 1968, Part III: The Records of the National Urban League, 1967–1979, box 2.

33. NUL, Synopsis of Statements of Concern, 1966 to 1971, July 1, 1972, Part III: The Records of the National Urban League, 1967–1979, Box 212.

34. NUL, Press Release, January 22, 1969, Part III: The Records of the National Urban League, 1967–1979, Box 189.

35. NUL, Workshop Reports, 1969 National Urban League Planning Conference, Tarrytown House, Tarrytown, N.Y., October 5, 1969, Part III: The Records of the National Urban League, 1967–1979, Box 284.

36. Ibid.

37. Ben A. Franklin, "Welfare Parley Cautious of Nixon," *New York Times,* August 24, 1969, 34.

38. NUL, Press Release, May 12, 1970, Part III: The Records of the National Urban League, 1967–1979, Box 327.

39. Ibid.

40. NUL, NUL Board of Trustees Meeting, November 18, 19, 1970, Part III: The Records of the National Urban League, 1967–1979, box 175.

41. NUL, Memo to: The Urban League Family, From: Whitney M. Young, Re: NUL Statement on Welfare Reform Legislation, December 4, 1970, Part III: The Records of the National Urban League, 1967–1979, Box 327.

42. C. Gerald Fraser, "Young Seeks Aid for Nation's Poor," *New York Times,* July 21, 1970, 1.

43. NUL, Draft—National Domestic Marshall Plan, July 1, 1970, Part III: The Records of the National Urban League, 1967–1979, Box 56.

44. NUL, Press Release, December 15, 1971, Part III: The Records of the National Urban League, 1967–1979, box 46.

45. NUL, Memo to: Vernon E. Jordan, Jr., From: Jeweldean J. Londa, Re: Current Public Assistance Crisis, October 22, 1971, Part III: The Records of the National Urban League, 1967–1979, Box 327.

46. NUL, Press Release: Urban League Opposes Welfare Bill, Jordan Tells

Senate Proposals Are Punitive, February 3, 1972, Part III: The Records of the National Urban League, 1967–1979, Box 46.

47. Alexander J. Allen, "Approaches to Welfare Reform," *New York Times*, March 3, 1972, 38.

48. NUL Executive Committee, March 17, 1972, Part III: The Records of the National Urban League, 1967–1979, Box 27.

49. NUL, An Address by Vernon E. Jordan, Executive Director, NUL at the NUL National Conference, July 30, 1972, Part III: The Records of the National Urban League, 1967–1979, Box 2.

50. NUL, Statement of Concern: Support for the National Welfare Rights Organization, August 2, 1972, Part III: The Records of the National Urban League, 1967–1979, Box 2.

Chapter 5. Explaining Priority Shifts During the 1960s

Epigraph: Letter to James Farmer from Jim Peck, November 30, 1965, CORE, Addendum, Subgroup A: National Director's Files, Series I, No. 20, Reel 1, Frame 384.

1. For personal accounts of fieldwork experience, see, for example, Forman 1997; Sellers 1990; Zinn 1965.

2. Many histories of civil rights organizations refer to this shift. For an analysis of changes for the movement overall to a focus on economic issues in general, see Hamilton and Hamilton 1997.

3. As Dawson 1994 argues, middle and upper class African Americans identify with lower-income blacks—therefore, even if civil rights groups consider the middle class to be their constituency, the organizations may be inclined to represent the interests of the black poor, particularly if the number of black poor increase, or if the proportion of African Americans living in poverty increases.

4. Scholars argue that poverty rates are not the most telling indicators of the overall economic position of African Americans. Income, wage, and wealth gaps are also used as indicators. Oliver and Shapiro (1989) argue that the wealth gap, a measure of net financial assets, between African Americans and whites is critical to assessing the life chances of African Americans. For the purposes of this study, however, I rely on poverty rates to determine whether civil rights leaders may have prioritized anti-poverty reform in response to dramatically increasing levels of poverty among African Americans. Based on my examination of historical archives and secondary organizational histories, I have found that leaders, boards of directors, and staff generally refer to poverty rates when discussing and assessing the socioeconomic position of African Americans. Additionally, an organization concerned with the wealth gap would not necessarily focus on anti-poverty policy, but would rather focus on economic policy more generally, and on the economic implications of employment and/or wage discrimination.

5. After the passage of the Social Security Act in 1935, recipients of ADC benefits, the precursor to AFDC, were overwhelmingly white. In 1937, 85 percent of the rolls were white, and 13 percent were black (Teles 1996, 24). Throughout the next three decades, this gap continued to shrink, until the percentages of recipients were almost equal during the 1960s, when each racial group comprised approximately 40 percent of recipients. The 1950s saw the most dramatic increase in the number of African Americans receiving assistance (Lieberman 1998, 168). Because southern aid offices were highly discriminatory in their practices, it was not until African Americans could apply for assistance

in the North that they began to receive it (Teles 1996, 26). It was not until the War on Poverty during the mid-1960s that welfare became associated with race for civil rights organizations, policy-makers, and those opposing the expansion of the welfare state (Lieberman 1998, 168). Before the War on Poverty, civil rights leaders were certainly aware of the link between race and poverty, and the disproportionate effect of poverty on African Americans, but policy-makers did not view policies intended to alleviate poverty as having any particular impact based on the race. In fact, during the period of policy formation for the War on Poverty, the Kennedy administration did not consider public aid to be an issue related to race (Patterson 2000, 129).

6. Other scholars also discuss the importance of issues to organizational decision-making. Browne (1998) assesses the attributes of issues in terms of whether they will bring success to an organization. He distinguishes between "good" and "bad" issues based on their appeal to policymakers, their social utility, and their relevance to multiple segments of the population, among other attributes. Not surprisingly, anti-poverty policy falls in Browne's "bad" policy category. Therefore, organizations have few incentives to make poverty a central priority.

7. On civil rights groups' ongoing engagement with economic issues, see Hamilton and Hamilton 1997.

8. NUL did receive substantial War on Poverty grants. However, it considered poverty a central priority before it began to receive federal funding; see Chapter 3.

9. See Chapter 3, also Table 5.1 in this chapter, for a reminder of trends in attention to anti-poverty policy among civil rights organizations.

10. In fact, the national office was consistently preoccupied with maintaining its control over local branches (Bracey and Meier 1997, v). Gloster B. Current, NAACP director of branches, emphasized the need to improve the national/local relationship throughout his career.

11. The NAACP has consistently been considered more conservative than other civil rights groups. On this reputation, and responding to it, see Bond in Jonas 2005; Smith in Johnson and Stanford 2002; Barker, Jones, and Tate 1999.

12. NAACP, Letter to Miss L. Pearl from Gloster B, Current, June 14, 1961, Supplement to Part XVI, Board of Directors File, 1956–1965, Group 3, Series A, Box 27.

13. NAACP, Report of the Secretary to the Board of Directors for the month of March, 1962, April 11, 1962, Supplement to Part I, 1960–1965, Group 3, Series A, Box A-31.

14. NAACP, Memo to John Morsell from Mildred Bond, Re: Staff Conference, March 12, 1960, Supplement to Part XVII, National Staff Files, 1956–1965, Group 3, Series A, Box A-307.

15. NAACP, Memo to John Morsell from Calvin D. Banks, Re: Reactions to Conference Proposals, March 12, 1960, Supplement to Part XVII, National Staff Files, 1956–1965, Group 3, Series A, Box A-307.

16. NAACP, Memo for Staff Conference, March 1960, from Herbert Hill, March 21, 1960, Supplement to Part XVII, National Staff Files, 1956–1965, Group 3, Series A, Box A-310.

17. NAACP, Memo to Presidents of Branches and State Conferences from Roy Wilkins, Re: Action Memo: NAACP in the War on Poverty, October 13, 1964, Supplement to Part XVII, National Staff Files, 1956–1965 Group 3, Series A, Box A-310.

18. NAACP, *NAACP Annual Convention Resolutions* 1965, Supplement to Part I, 1960–1965, Group 3, Series A, Box A-20.

19. NAACP, Memo to Mr. Roy Wilkins, From: Richard W. McClain, ADMINIS-TRATIVELY CONFIDENTIAL, Part IV, Box 90, July 26, 1967; Memo to Wilkins; Thru: Richard McClain, Robert Saunders, Virna Canson, FROM: Maurice Dawkins, RE: A policy for NAACP member participation in non profit neighborhood economic development corporation, July 20, 1967, Part IV, Box 90.

20. NAACP, Board of Directors Meeting Minutes, April 12, 1965, Supplement to Part I, 1960–1965, Group 3, Series A, Box A-26.

21. NUL, Board Meeting Minutes, May 21, 1964, Part III: The Records of the National Urban League, 1967–1979, Box 170,.

22. NUL, Press Release, May 24, 1965, Part II: The Records of the National Urban League, 1960–1966, Series V, Box 35.

23. NUL, Memo to Young, From: Evelyn Broidy, Re: Poverty Workshop—Birmingham, AL, February 26–27, March 5, 1965, Part II: The Records of the National Urban League, 1960–1966, Series I, Box 42; also see NUL, "Agenda for the Future," Address by Whitney Young, 55th Annual Conference, August 1, 1965, Part II: The Records of the National Urban League, 1960–1966, Series VI, Box 20.

24. NUL, Memo to: Annual Delegate Assembly, From: Henry Steeger, NUL President, Re: Policy Statement on Non-Violent Techniques, July 19, 1963, Part II: The Records of the National Urban League, 1960–1966, Series I, Box 28.

25. NUL, Press Release, June 29, 1965, Part II: The Records of the National Urban League, 1960–1966, Series V, Box 35.

26. Ibid.

27. NUL, Board Meeting Minutes, November 19, 1963, Part III: The Records of the National Urban League, 1967–1979, Box 170.

28. NUL, Press Release, April 9, 1964, Part II: The Records of the National Urban League, 1960–1966, Series I, Box 27.

29. NUL, Board Meeting Minutes, August 2, 1965, Part III: The Records of the National Urban League, 1967–1979, Box 170.

30. NUL, Press Release, April 9, 1964.

31. NUL, Summary Report of the 1964 National Conference, Poverty Reexamined: Old Problems, New Challenges, August 1, 1964, Part II: The Records of the National Urban League, 1960–1966, Series IV, Box 21.

32. NUL, "Summary and Recommendations: NUL War on Poverty Workshop," May 20, 1964, Part II: The Records of the National Urban League, 1960–1966, Series I, Box 38.

33. SNCC, Minutes of SNCC Regional Meeting, March 24, 1962, Subgroup A, Atlanta Office, 1959–1972, Series III: Staff Meetings, 1960–1968, Reel 3, Frame 806.

34. SNCC, Minutes of the SNCC Executive Committee Meeting, December 27, 1963, Subgroup A, Atlanta Office, 1959–1972, Series II: Executive and Central Committees, 1961–1967, Reel 3, Frame 329.

35. SNCC, Memo to SNCC Executive Committee from Eleanor Holmes, re: SNCC and the Big 10 of the March on Washington, September 6, 1963, Subgroup A, Atlanta Office, 1959–1972, Series II: Executive and Central Committees, 1961–1967, Reel 3, Frame 275.

36. SNCC, Some Comments on the Civil Rights Movement, Reprinted from the NY Herald Tribune, by John Lewis, May 23, 1965, Subgroup A, Atlanta Office, 1959–1972, Series VII: Communications Department, 1960–1968, Reel 14, Frame 329.

37. SNCC, Minutes of SNCC regional meeting—Atlanta, March 24, 1962, 6.

38. Ibid.

39. SNCC, Minutes of June Meeting of the Coordinating Committee, June 1–2, 1962, Subgroup A, Atlanta Office, 1959–1972, Series V: SNCC Conferences, 1960–1964, Reel 11, Frame 813.

40. SNCC, Memo to SNCC Executive Committee from Eleanor Holmes, September 6, 1963, Subgroup A, Atlanta Office, 1959–1972, Series II: Executive and Central Committees, 1961–1967, Reel 3, Frame 275.

41. CORE, Amended Constitution of CORE, March 1958, Series I: National Director's File, No. 21, Reel 2, Frame 301.

42. CORE, "Some Remarks on the 1960 CORE Convention," by James R. Robinson, July 20, 1960, Series III: Executive Secretary's File, No. 23, Reel 2, Frame 537.

43. CORE, "The Control of National CORE," June 1, 1961, Series IV: National Action Council, No. 1, Reel 16, Frame 440, emphasis in original.

44. CORE, 22nd Annual Convention, National Director's Report, Addendum, Subgroup C: National Action Council and Conventions, July 2, 1964, No. 80, Reel 9, Frame 786.

45. CORE, Memo to Field Secretaries from James T. McCain, Director, Re: Servicing Chapters, Procedures for Setting Up New Chapters, Affiliation, Organizing in New Areas, Communication between Staff, chapters, and national office, March 24, 1964, Series V: Departments and Related Organizations, No. 293, Reel 38, Frame 925.

46. CORE, Memo to: Contact List, From: Norman Hill/Program Director, Re: Proposed Educational Series for Chapters, December 1, 1963, Series I: National Director's Files, No. 25, Reel 2, Frame 761.

47. CORE, By-Laws of CORE, as compiled by the NAC, June 19, 1964, Series I: National Director's File, No. 23, Reel 2, Frame 577.

48. CORE, NAACP Meeting—December 31, 1965–January 2, 1966, Addendum, subgroup C: National Action Council and Conventions, no. 1, Reel 107, Frame 992.

49. On CORE's decline and chapter activities during the late 1960s, see Meier and Rudwick 1975 [1973], 357–73.

50. CORE, Letter to Mrs. James L. Davis from Herbert Callender, Director of Organization, May 12, 1966, Addendum, Subgroup F, Organization Department, Series I, No. 27, Reel 16, Frame 897.

51. CORE, Open Session: Recommendation of Statement—War on Poverty or War in Vietnam, January 1966, Addendum, Subgroup C, National Action Council and Conventions, Series I, No. 107, Reel 9, Frame 995.

52. CORE, Memo, CONFIDENTIAL, To: Department Heads, Re: Minutes of Staff Meeting, May 15, 1967, Addendum, Subgroup A, National Director's Files, Series II, No. 95, Reel 6, Frame 1047.

53. CORE, Political Action on the Community Level: Part I," by Karin Berg, Staff Associate, July 1, 1965, Addendum, Subgroup A, National Directors' Files, Series I, No. 80, Reel 2, Frame 80.

54. CORE, "Community Organization" Discussion Outline, CORE Summer Project Orientation, June 1965, Series V: Departments and Related Organizations, No. 132, Reel 26, Frame 492.

55. See Garrow 1986; Fairclough 1987; Peake 1987.

56. See Morris 1984; Peake 1987.

57. SCLC, Memo to King from R. T. Blackwell, January 27, 1966, Part 3, Reel 3, Box 45.

58. SCLC, Constitution and By-Laws of the SCLC, Part 2, Reel 1, Subgroup 2, 1957.

59. SCLC, "These are the broad areas of concern, agreed upon by committee on resolution, to be developed and refined for public relations purposes," Part 2, Reel 1, Subgroup 2, 1957.

60. SCLC, "Operation Breadbasket—organizational flyer," Part 4, Reel 23, Box 172, 1963.

61. SCLC, Constitution and By-Laws of the SCLC, *Records of the Southern Christian Leadership Conference, 1954–1970, Part 2: Records of the Executive Director and Treasurer,* Reel 1, Subgroup 2, 1957.

62. SCLC, "Staff Report: The Washington Bureau," Part 4, Reel 8, Box 146, 1964.

63. SCLC, "SCLC: Resolutions" Part 3, Reel 7, Box 128, 1965.

64. SCLC, "Rationale and Budget for Southern Christian Leadership Conference Department of Affiliates," Part 2, Reel 22, Subgroup 3, 1965.

65. Bernard LaFayette, Interview with author, July 10, 2008.

66. SCLC, Press Release: Dr. King Announces Complete Reorganization of SCLC and Appointment of Three Executives, Part 3, Reel 4, 1967.

Chapter 6. Explaining Priority Shifts During the Early 1970s

1. I have chosen to discuss the factors that led to declining levels of NAACP and NUL attention between the late 1960s and early 1970s because it is the only legislative period in which more than one organization decreased its attention to anti-poverty policy at the national level, with the exception of the NAACP and SNCC between the War on Poverty and the late 1960s (see Figure 5.1). I have chosen not to highlight this period of decline because, for SNCC, the decrease in attention to anti-poverty policy was caused by the organization's overall decline during the period. It would be difficult to find any issue area of national priority tied to national legislation for SNCC between the mid- and late 1960s. Therefore, an examination of the factors that led to SNCC's decreasing attention to anti-poverty policy would not be particularly meaningful, except to point to the organization's overall decline. SNCC staff dropped from 150 in 1967 to 78 in 1970. The organization's income dropped from $637,736 in 1969 to $25,000 in 1970. On staff numbers in 1965 see SNCC Letter to Supporters, November 1, 1965, Subgroup A, Atlanta Office, 1959–1972, Series I: Chairman's Files 1960–1969; on staff numbers in 1967 see Staff List, March 1967, Subgroup C, Washington Office, 1960–1968, Series II: Subject Files, 1963–1968. Organization's income for all years from Haines 1998, 84.

2. Francis E. Ward, "Dearth of Leadership in Civil Rights Grows," *Los Angeles Times,* April 22, 1971, 16.

3. Vernon Jarett, "The NAACP Stands on a Proud Record," *Chicago Tribune,* February 11, 1972, 18.

4. NAACP, Louis Harris Survey for *Newsweek,* Summary report by NAACP, Part IV, Box A85.

5. Gallup Organization, conducted for *Newsweek,* Survey of national adult blacks, May 1969.

6. Francis Ward, "Urban League Adopts More Militant stance," *Los Angeles Times,* August 10, 1971, A14.

7. Wilkins 1994 [1982], 319.

8. NAACP, 60th Annual Convention Resolutions, July 1, 1969, Part IX: Washington Bureau, Box 10.

9. NAACP, Convention Resolutions, 1970, July 11, 1970, Part VIII: 1965–1999, Box 1.

10. NAACP, Roy Innis, "The NAACP: Outdated and Outmoded," *Manhattan Tribune*, November 28, 1970, Part IX, Washington Bureau, Box 155.

11. NAACP, Letter to the Editor, *Manhattan Tribune*, from John A. Morsell, Assistant Executive Director, NAACP, December 10, 1970, Part IX: Washington Bureau, Box 155.

12. On CORE's organizational weakness by 1968, see Meier and Rudwick 1975 [1973], 425; on SNCC's decline see Carson 1995, 295.

13. Wilkins 1994 [1982], 319.

14. NAACP, Letter to Whitney Young from Roy Wilkins, August 3, 1970, Part VIII: 1965–1999, Box 368.

15. On the NUL shift to militancy, see Francis Ward, "Urban League Adopts More Militant stance," *Los Angeles Times*, August 10, 1971, A14.

16. NAACP, Remarks of Roy Wilkins, Executive Director, at the Annual Membership Meeting of the NAACP, January 10, 1972, Part VIII: 1965–1999, Box 61.

17. NAACP, *Annual Report 1970*, January 1971.

18. NAACP, Report to the 63rd Annual Convention from the national board of the question of term and tenure of national board members, July 1, 1972, Part VIII: 1965–1999, Box 61.

19. Foundations gave to the NAACP each year; only NUL consistently received more foundation funding. Based on giving from the Ford and Rockefeller Foundations and Carnegie Corporation, foundation funding comprised 2–4 percent of total NAACP income between 1967 and 1974, with the exception of 1970, when foundation funding comprised 8 percent. Source: Foundation giving: Marger 1984, 25; calculations of percentage of total income by author based on the NAACP *Annual Report.*

20. "Ford Foundation Gives the NAACP $300,000 Again," *Chicago Daily Defender*, July 19, 1969, 5.

21. NAACP, NAACP Board of Directors Meeting, July 4, 1969, Part VIII: 1965–1999, Box 61.

22. "NAACP Hikes Members Fees," *Chicago Daily Defender*, July 19, 1969.

23. NAACP, Letter to Branch Officers from Gloster Current and Lucille Black, Secretary for Membership, July 13, 1970, Part VIII: 1965–1999, Box 10.

24. NAACP, *Annual Report 1972*, January 1973.

25. See NAACP, Quarterly Report to the Washington Bureau, September 3, 1970, Part VIII: 1965–1999, Box 61; Statement of Clarence Mitchell, Director of the Washington Bureau and Legislative Chairman of the LCCR before the House Committee on Education and Labor on OEO Legislation, March 31, 1971, Part IX: Washington Bureau, Box 169.

26. See Figure 5.4 for levels of foundation funding to NUL between 1967 and 1974. Foundation funding spiked in 1970, and then dropped substantially by 1971, the year when federal funding of NUL New Thrust programming began.

27. NUL, A New Thrust for the Urban League Movement, June 5, 1968, Part III: The Records of the National Urban League, 1967–1979, Box 35.

28. NUL, "Building Ghetto Power," Speeches Presented at the 58th Annual NUL Conference, New Orleans, July 28–August 1, 1968, Part III: The Records of the National Urban League, 1967–1979, Box 2.

29. NUL, 1969–1970 A Discussion Prospectus, September 17, 1969, Part III: The Records of the National Urban League, 1967–1979, Box 361.

30. Ibid.

31. Between 1967 and 1970, foundation funding to NUL increased from just under $1 million to just under $5 million. Real dollar amounts (in 2002 dollars) calculated by author based on nominal dollar amounts in Marger 1984, 25.

32. Rudy Johnson, "Whitney Young Scores Nixon's Policy," *New York Times*, July 29, 1969.

33. Ethel L. Payne, "Young Says He Hasn't Written Off Nixon Yet," *Chicago Daily Defender*, August 9, 1969, 6.

34. C. Gerald Fraser, "Negro Coalition to Meet White Urged by Young," *New York Times*, July 20, 1970.

35. NUL, National Urban League, Progress Report, 1971, January 1972, Part III: The Records of the National Urban League, 1967–1979, Box 14.

36. NUL, Report by Harold R. Sims before the 1971 NUL Delegate Assembly, July 28, 1971, Part III: The Records of the National Urban League, 1967–1979, Box 212.

37. NUL, Letter to Young from Frank Carlucci, Acting Director, OEO, January 12, 1971, Part III: The Records of the National Urban League, 1967–1979, Box 233.

38. NUL, Memo to: Cabinet Members, From: M. Leo Bohanon, August 4, 1971, Part III: The Records of the National Urban League, 1967–1979, Box 207.

39. NUL, Report by Harold R. Sims before 1971 NUL Delegate Assembly, July 28, 1971.

40. NUL, Address by Vernon E. Jordan, Jr., Executive Director Designate, 1971 NUL Conference, July 28, 1971, Part III: The Records of the National Urban League, 1967–1979, Box 2.

41. NUL, Letter to Young from the Ford Foundation, October 4, 1968, Part III: The Records of the National Urban League, 1967–1979, Box 60.

42. NUL, 1969–1970 Discussion Prospectus.

43. NUL, A New Thrust for the Urban League Movement: Operations Manual, July 17, 1968, Part II: The Records of the National Urban League, 1960–1966, Box 35.

44. NUL, 1968 NUL Staff Retreat, Tarrytown House, Tarrytown, NY, October 5, 1968, Morning Session, Part III: The Records of the National Urban League, 1967–1979, Box 284.

45. NUL, Memo to: NUL Cabinet Members, From: Sterling Tucker, Re: Summary of Tarrytown Conference and Next Steps, October 15, 1970, Part III: The Records of the National Urban League, 1967–1979, Box 284.

46. NUL, Memo to: Members of the Ad Hoc Planning Unit Task Force, From: Sterling Tucker, Central Planning Unit Coordinator, Re: Purpose and Scope of Task Force Meetings, February 10–12, 1971. February 3, 1971, Part III: The Records of the National Urban League, 1967–1979, Box 184.

47. NUL, Memo to: Cabinet Members, From: M. Leo Bohanon, August 4, 1971.

48. Ibid.

49. NUL, National Urban League: Terms of Affiliation for Urban League Affiliates, July 28, 1971, Part III: The Records of the National Urban League, 1967–1979, Box 237.

50. NUL, Memo to Harold R. Sims, Acting Executive Director, From: Sterling Tucker, March 30, 1971, Part III: The Records of the National Urban League, 1967–1979, Box 184.

51. Ibid.

52. NUL, "The First Six Months," Report of the Department of Government Affairs, National Urban League, July 1, 1972, Part III: The Records of the National Urban League, 1967–1979.

53. NUL, Memo to: Members of the Ad Hoc Planning Unit Task Force.

Chapter 7. Recent Battles, Recent Challenges

Epigraphs: Julian Bond, chairman of NAACP National Board of Directors, Remarks at 98th Annual NAACP Convention, July 8, 2007, Cobo Hall, Detroit; Hugh B. Price, National Urban League president and CEO, interview with author, July 8, 2009.

1. On the importance of organizational archives to assessing reasons for behavior, see Appendix A.

2. Advocacy groups, including the Children's Defense Fund and NOW, were very active concerning TANF reform (Weaver 2000). However, neither group's primary mission is to advocate on behalf of the poor; both organizations are Washington-based groups engaged in mainstream lobbying.

3. Mink 1998 argues that another purpose of the legislation was to control childbearing among African American women; see also Hancock 2004.

4. See Weaver 2000 for a discussion of interest groups engaged in battles on the 1996 legislation, noting the absence of organizations representing welfare recipients. Active organizations included intergovernmental lobbying organizations, such as the National Governors Association, Center for Budget and Policy Priorities, Center for Law and Social Policy, Children's Defense Fund, and social conservative organizations such as the Christian Coalition (197).

5. Congressional Quarterly 1996, 7–39. Also see Mink 1999, 1998 on the bipartisan consensus that led to the 1996 reforms.

6. See Hamilton and Hamilton 1997 for a discussion of civil rights organizations' opposition to the bases of welfare reform during 1994 and 1996.

7. Jeff Gammage, "NAACP Reexamines Its Mission/Bouncing Back from Debt and Scandal, the Group Seeks to Redefine Itself," *Philadelphia Inquirer,* July 14, 1997, A01.

8. David Hatchett, "Lives in the Balance: The New Welfare Reform," *The Crisis* 102, 2 (February/March 2005).

9. Hugh B. Price, Interview with author, New Rochelle, N.Y., July 8, 2009.

10. "Homelessness in Black America," *The Crisis* 102, 8 (November/December 1995): 14.

11. Elsa Brenner, "NAACP Chapters See More Work Ahead," *New York Times,* April 23, 1995, 1.

12. NAACP, Press Release, "New NAACP Chief Vows Activism/Myrlie-Evers Williams said Congress' Views Challenge Us on a Daily Basis," February 20, 1995.

13. Michael A. Fletcher, "Low-Profile Year 'Extremely Productive' for NAACP, Mfume Says," *Washington Post,* February 16, 1997, A03.

14. Ibid.

15. Gammage, "NAACP Reexamines Its Mission."

16. Price, interview with author.

17. NUL, *The State of Black America 1995* (New York: National Urban League, 1995), 2.

18. Price, interview with author.

19. NUL, *The State of Black America 1995,* 2

20. Price, interview with author.

21. NUL, *The State of Black America 1996* (New York: National Urban League, 1966), 9–10.

22. Price, interview with author.

23. Cheryl Wetzstein, "Sides See Welfare Reform Signing Near; Gingrich Expects President's OK," *Washington Times*, July 30, 1996, A7.

24. Hugh Price, quoted in "Parties at Crossroads on Helping the Poor," *Philadelphia Inquirer*, August 18, 1996, E01.

25. NUL, *1997 Annual Report*, January 1998, 4.

26. NUL, *1997 Annual Report*, 5.

27. See CNN, "Special Reports: Hurricane Katrina," for a detailed timeline of Katrina's progress and federal, state, and local responses, http://www.cnn.com/SPECIALS/2005/katrina/, accessed April 3, 2009.

28. Manning Marable, "Introduction," in Marable and Clarke 2008, 3–16.

29. Dara Strolovitch, Dorian Warren, and Paul Frymer, "Katrina's Political Roots and Divisions: Race, Class, and Federalism in American Politics," Social Science Research Council, June 11, 2006, http://www.understandingkatrina.ssrc.org/FrymerStrolovitchWarren/, accessed March 7, 2009. Also see Frymer, Strolovtich, and Warren 2006.

30. For a timeline of legislative and executive actions in response to Katrina, see Matt Fellowes and Amy Liu, "Federal Allocations in Response to Katrina, Rita, and Wilma: An Update," August 21, 2006, http://www.brookings.edu/~/media/Files/rc/reports/2006/08metropolitanpolicy_fellowes/20060712_Katrinafactsheet.pdf, accessed April 29, 2009.

31. On the "discovery" of American poverty during Katrina, see Dyson 2007; Childs 2007.

32. Marable, "Introduction."

33. Nicole Barnes 2005 "Mississippi State NAACP Responds to the Needs of Katrina Victims," *The Crisis* 112, 6 (November/December 2005): 57.

34. NAACP, *2005 Annual Report*, January 2006, 5.

35. Amanda S. Miller, "NAACP Partners with Habitat for Humanity to Build Gulf Coast Homes," *The Crisis* (March/April 2006): 50.

50. Also see NAACP, *2005 Annual Report*, January 2006.

36. NAACP Press Release, "NAACP Hollywood Bureau in the Community," n.d., http://www.naacp.org/programs/hollywood/community/index.htm, accessed May 15, 2009.

37. Michael Fletcher, "Black Leaders Respond to Katrina Disaster," *The Crisis* 112, 6 (November/December 2005): 10.

38. William E. Spriggs, "Poverty in America: The Poor Are Getting Poorer," *The Crisis* (January/February 2006): 14–19.

39. "Remembering Hurricane Katrina: NAACP Focuses on Housing in the Gulf Coast Region One Year Later," *NAACP Advocate: A Publication of the Research, Advocacy and Training Division* 1, 3 (September 2006): 1.

40. Wanda Davis, "Now Homeless, a Mother Recounts Katrina," *The Crisis* (September/October 2006): 48.

41. NAACP Policies in Welfare, 2007, www.naacp.com, accessed May 2009.

42. Lottie L. Joiner, "NAACP Offers Assistance to Displaced Voters in New Orleans Election," *The Crisis* 113, 3 (May/June 2006): 60.

43. "National Legislative Priorities for the 109th Congress," June 6, 2008, http://www.naacp.org/about/resources/manuals/109th_legislative_priorities.pdf, accessed May 12, 2009.

44. "NAACP Legislative Priorities for the 109thCongress—Full Explana-

tions," June 6, 2006, http://www.naacp.org/about/resources/manuals/109th
_legislative...priorities.pdf, accessed May 12, 2009.

45. Frankie Gamber, "NAACP Helps Thousands of Katrina Victims with Housing, Food, and Care," *The Crisis* 112, 6 (November/December 2005): 56.

46. Ibid..

47. Frankie Gamber, "Baton Rouge Police Accused of Abuse After Katrina," *The Crisis* (January/February 2006): 55.

48. Frankie Gamber, "NAACP Remembers Hurricane Victims in Alabama," *The Crisis* (November/December 2006): 60.

49. Nicole Barnes, "Mississippi State NAACP Responds to the Needs of Katrina Victims," *The Crisis* 112, 6 (November/December 2005): 57.

50. Nedra Lindsey, "NAACP Appoints Director of New Orleans Katrina Relief Center," *The Crisis* (July/August 2006).

51. "Remembering Hurricane Katrina," 1.

52. Iris Raeshaun, "One Year After Hurricane Katrina, Housing Shortage Persists in Gulf," *The Crisis* (November/December 2006): 58.

53. On Gordon's resignation, see Raymond Hernandez, "Chief Leaving After Brief Stay at NAACP," *New York Times*, March 4, 2007, A01. On organizational turmoil and "right-sizing," see Bond, Remarks at 98th Annual NAACP Convention.

54. Press Release: "On Second Anniversary, Government Assistance to Hurricane Evacuees and Recovery Is Woefully Lacking," August 29, 2007, http://www.naacp.org/news/press/2007–08–29/index.htm, accessed May 18, 2009.

55. "Don't Let Congress Forget Them Again," April 24, 2007, http://www.naacp.org/about/leadership/directors/chaircorner/2007–08–24-katrina/index.htm, accessed May 18, 2009.

56. Press Release, "NAACP urges Congress to pass post-Katrina employment, rebuild, and development legislation before September congressional adjournment," September 15, 2008, http://www.naacp.org/news/press/2008–15–08/index.htm, accessed April 13, 2008.

57. "NAACP Platform Analysis 2008 Election," August 1, 2008, http://www.naacp.org/programs/bureau-dc/2008.Platform.Comparison.color.pdf, accessed April 15, 2009.

58. Bond, Remarks at 98th Annual NAACP Convention.

59. "NAACP Opposed Bush's 2009 Budget Proposal; White House Would Eliminate and/or Cripple Many Crucial Domestic Services and Programs While Benefitting the Wealthiest Americans," March 11, 2008, http://www.naacp.org/get-involved/activism/alerts/110thaa-2008–03–11/index.htm, accessed on April 30, 2009.

60. Press Release, "Mississippi President Testifies Before Congressional Committee on Federal Housing Funds for Hurricane Katrina Survivors," May 8, 2008, http://www.naacp.org/news/press/2008–05–08/index.htm, accessed May 17, 2009.

61. Press Release, "As New Storms Rise, NAACP Calls for Continued Focus and Support for Those Still Rebuilding Lives Three Years After Katrina," August 29, 2008, http://www.naacp.org/news/press/2008–08–29/index.htm, accessed February 19, 2009.

62. Press Release, "Louisiana NAACP Continues Efforts to Assist Katrina Victims," April 25, 2007, http://www.naacp.org/news/press/2007–04–25–2/index.htm, accessed May 9, 2009.

63. DeShuna Spencer, "NAACP Fights for Gulf Coast Residents," *The Crisis* (May/June 2007): 42.

64. Press Release, "On Second Anniversary."
65. Press Release, "BET, National Urban League, American Red Cross to Announce Prime Time Telethon to Benefit Hurricane Katrina Victims," August 31, 2005, http://www.nul.org/ Publications/telethon.pdf, accessed May 16, 2009.
66. NUL, *2005 Annual Report,* January 2006, http://www.nul.org/publica tions/AnnualReport/2005AnnualRpt.pdf, accessed May 14, 2009.
67. Ibid.
68. Press Release, "National Urban League Calls for a 'Katrina Bill of Rights,'" September 8, 2005, http://www.nul.org/PressReleases/2005/2005 PR222.html, accessed February 21, 2009.
69. Ibid.
70. NUL, *2005 Annual Report.*
71. Ibid., 3.
72. Press Release, "National Urban League President and CEO Marc Morial Questions New Orleans Recovery Plan," January 7, 2006, http://www.nul.org/ PressReleases/2006/2006pr305.html, accessed May 15, 2009.
73. Press Release, "National Urban League President Marc Morial Calls for Immediate Inspection of Nation's Flood Control to Avert Katrina Repeat," May 23, 2006, http://www.nul.org/PressReleases/2006/2006pr329.html, accessed May 16, 2009.
74. Ibid.
75. Press Release, "National Urban League Says Rebuild New Orleans Plan Violates Katrina Victims' Right to Return," January 11, 2006, http://www.nul .org/PressReleases/2006/ 2006pr307.html, accessed May 15, 2009.
76. Press Release, "National Urban League President Marc Morial Demands That Secretary Michael Chertoff Rescind Order and Keep Promise Not to Kick Out Katrina Evacuees," April 27, 2006, http://www.nul.org/PressReleases/ 2006/2006pr324.html, accessed May 16, 2009.
77. NUL, *Katrina: One Year Later: A Policy and Research Report on the National Urban League's Katrina Bill of Rights* (New York: National Urban League, 2006), 3–4.
78. Press Release, "Recovery Less Than Impressive One Year After Katrina, Urban League Report Shows," August 24, 2006, http://www.nul.org/Press Releases/2006/2006pr360.html, accessed April 21, 2009.
79. Ibid.
80. Press Release, "National Urban League Continues Fight to Help Hurricane Katrina Survivors Recover," August 29, 2007, http://www.nul.org/Press Releases/2007/2007pr418.html, accessed on February 22, 2009.
81. Marc Morial, "To Be Equal: Katrina Recovery in Major Need of National Summit to Get the Job Done for Once and for All," February 1, 2007, http:// www.nul.org/publications/TBE/2007/TBE-COL-05.pdf, accessed March 3, 2009.
82. Marc H. Morial, "House Gulf Coast Recovery Bill Stands Little Chance of Becoming Law," *Bay State Banner,* April 5, 2007.
83. Morial, "To Be Equal: Politics as Usual?"
84. Press Release, "National Urban League Continues Fight.
85. Marc Morial, "To Be Equal: Hurricane Recovery Legislation Would Give Katrina Survivors Permanent Shelter, Peace of Mind," November 7, 2007, http://www.nul.org/publications/TBE/2007/TBE-COL-44.pdf, accessed April 1, 2009.

86. Marc Morial, "To Be Equal: Remember Katrina," May 21, 2008, http://www.nul.org/publications/TBE/2008/TBE-COL-17.pdf, accessed March 23, 2009.

87. Marc Morial, "To Be Equal: Fix the Levees Now," September 17, 2008, http://www.nul.org/publications/TBE/2008/TBE-COL-33.pdf, accessed March 23, 2009.

88. NUL, *2005 Annual Report.*

Conclusions

1. The tension between economic and political concerns during field organizing in the 1960s is well documented; see Carson 1995; Meier and Rudwick 1975 [1973]; Ransby 2003; D'Emilio 2003. For personal accounts of field experience, see, for example, Forman 1997; Sellers 1990; Zinn 1965.

2. Particularly in discussions of poverty and race, it may be tempting to argue that civil rights organizations advocate on behalf of the poor because they are ideologically driven to do so. Not surprisingly, scholars have argued that members of civil rights organizations are particularly ideologically driven concerning issues of racial equality (Wilson 1995 [1973]; Bayes 1982). The findings in this project indicate that ideological commitment to either racial or economic equity does not determine the level of attention an organization devotes to anti-poverty policy.

3. On the expansion of gay and lesbian organizations' outreach to transgendered organizations and individuals, see Eaklor 2004; D'Emilio 2004.

4. On the history of transgendered grassroots organizations and activism, see Jones 2004; Feinberg 1996.

5. On the obstacles faced by organizations representing the poor, see Hays 2001; Piven and Cloward 1977; Walker 1991; Berry and Arons 2003.

6. See Appendix B for tables of magnitude change.

7. On civil rights organizations' concern with economic issues, see Hamilton and Hamilton 1997.

8. See Dawson 1994 on notions of linked racial fate among African Americans. On common policy interests among low- and middle-income African Americans, see Pattillo-McCoy 1999 .

9. See Hays 2001; Piven and Cloward 1971.

10. On lack of representation of the poor, see Chapter 1; also Strolovitch 2007; Berry 2003; Rosenstone and Hansen 1993; Walker 1991; Schattschneider 1960; Verba, Schlozman, and Brady 1997.

11. Dawson's (1994) findings that middle-class African Americans share concerns, and have substantial contact, with low-income African Americans support the notion that civil rights organizations would be more inclined than other groups to advocate on behalf of the poor.

Appendix A: Archival Research and Coding

1. NAACP, Supplement to Part 17: National Staff Files, Reel 4, Frame 770.

2. For the microfilmed collections, the time reported is very approximate. Because I did not need to travel extensively to view the microfilm, I researched in the library for several hours each day. The length of time spent with the

microfilmed collections does not reflect whole weeks devoted to research, as it would on a research trip.

3. This explanation of the size and content of the collections is based on information in the guides to both collections: *The Papers of the Congress of Racial Equality, 1941–1967: A Guide to the Microfilm Collection* (Sanford, N.C.; Microfilming Corporation of America, 1980); *The Papers of the Congress of Racial Equality: Addendum 1944–1980* (Ann Arbor, Mich.: University Microfilms, 1982).

4. *Papers Guide*, 3–4.

5. *Addendum Guide*, 5.

6. *Addendum Guide*, 5.

7. Although I ended up using data only through 1973, I researched NAACP files through the late 1980s. Therefore, I received permission before my trip to the Library of Congress. The Library coordinates this process, and requests permission for researchers from the organization. The process can be lengthy—a researcher should apply for permission months, not weeks, before a visit.

8. "Supplement" refers to the date of the materials. Part I of the collection includes the Meetings of the Board of Directors, Records of Annual Conferences, Major Speeches, and Special Reports between 1909 and 1950. The Supplement I examined includes 1961–1965.

9. *Papers of the NAACP, Supplement to Part 17: National Staff Files, Guide*, John H. Bracey, Jr., and August Meier, General Editors (Frederick, Md.: University Publications of America, 1996).

10. *National Association for the Advancement of Colored People, Part IV, A Register of Its Records at the Library of Congress*, prepared by Joseph Sullivan, Manuscript Division, Library of Congress, Washington, D.C., 1996.

11. *National Association for the Advancement of Colored People, Part VII, A Register of Its Records at the Library of Congress*, prepared by Joseph K. Brooks, Manuscript Division, Library of Congress, Washington, D.C., 2000.

12. *National Association for the Advancement of Colored People, Part VIII, A Register of Its Records at the Library of Congress*, prepared by Melinda K. Friend, Margaret McAleer, and Michael Spangler, Manuscript Division, Library of Congress, Washington, D.C., 2000.

13. *National Association for the Advancement of Colored People, Part IX, A Register of Its Records at the Library of Congress*, prepared by Joseph K. Brooks and Michael Spangler, Manuscript Division, Library of Congress, Washington, D.C., 1997.

14. A container is a small file box, holding approximately 15 file folders.

15. *National Urban League: A Register of Its Records in the Library of Congress, Part III*, prepared by Harry G. Heiss, 1993.

16. *National Urban League, Office of Washington Operations, a Register of Its Records in the Library of Congress, Part I*, prepared by Joseph D. Sullivan; *Part II*, prepared by Harry G. Heiss, 1994.

17. *The Student Nonviolent Coordinating Committee Papers, 1959–1972: A Guide to the Microfilm Edition* (Sanford, N.C.: Microfilming Corporation of America, 1982), 2.

18. *The Student Nonviolent Coordinating Committee Papers, 1959–1972*, 4.

19. *Records of the Southern Christian Leadership Conference, 1954–1970*, Guides to Parts 1–4. Guide compiled by Blair Hydrick (Bethesda, Md.: University Publications of America, 2005).

20. I created databases using Filemaker Pro.

21. The "folder" field refers to the location of the document in my files.

22. Importantly, the number of documents I collected from each archive does not necessarily correlate with the size of the archive. I collected the most documents from the CORE archives because the organization was experiencing rapid growth and expansion in the South. Therefore, its archives from the 1960s hold extensive debates concerning, and documentation of, the organization's structure. Additionally, local offices were particularly active concerning anti-poverty policy. The NAACP and NUL archives include more documents, but CORE produced more documents relevant to my research during the periods I examined.

Figure 5.2. *Poverty rates*: U.S. Census Bureau, "Historical Poverty Tables," www
.census.gov/hhes/poverty/histpov, accessed January 3, 2004. *AFDC receipt*: 1960:
Piven and Cloward 1993 [1971], 194; 1969–1979: U.S. House Committee on
Ways and Means, Background Material and Data on Programs within the Jurisdiction of the Committee, 1988 ed., March 24, 1988.

Figure 5.3. NAACP Annual Reports, 1960–1968.

Figure 5.4. *Income source*: 1961: NUL, Part II, Records of the National Urban
League, 1960–1966, Series I, Box 27, Financial Statement, 1963; 1962 and 1963,
NUL Annual Reports; 1964: NUL, Part II, Series I, Box 2, Memo to William R.
Simms and John J. Garra, From: ZC McAdams, Re: Income for Source January–
September 1964, 1963, October 6, 1964; 1965 and 1966: author's estimate based
on income trend; 1967: NUL Annual Report. *Chapters source*: 1961–1967: NUL,
Part III, Records, 1967–1979, Box 48, Number Full-Time Employees in Urban
League 1961–1967; 1968: NUL, Part III, Box 2, Whitney Young, Address at the
1970 Annual Conference, "Building Ghetto Power"

Figure 5.5. *Adjusted income source*: Haines 1988, 84. *Staff source*: 1961: Stoper
1989, 71; 1962, 1964: SNCC, Subgroup A: Atlanta Office, 1959–1972, Series II:
Executive and Central Committees, 1961–1967, Memo to all SNCC Project
Heads from the Executive Committee of SNCC, February 24, 1964, Reel 3,
Frame 280; 1963: SNCC, Subgroup A, Series II, Letter to Barbara Miller c/o
Avedon, December 10, 1963; 1965: SNCC, Subgroup A, Series II, Letter to Sup-
porters, December 1965; 1966: SNCC, Subgroup A, Series II, Staff List, May
1966; 1967: SNCC, Subgroup A, Series II, Staff List, March 1967.

Figure 5.6. *Staff source*: 1958: Executive Secretary's report to 1958 CORE Convention, n.d., Series IV: National Action Council, No. 1, Reel 16, Frame 559;
1959, 1964: Rich 1965; 1960: Special Steering Committee Meeting, January 15,
1965; 1960–1963: Series IV: National Action Council, No. 1, Reel 1, Frame 1032;
1965: "CORE National Office," October 22, 1965, B: Associate National Director's Files, Series I, No. 40, Reel 9, Frame 218. *Chapters source*: 1958, 1959: Meier

and Rudwick 1973, 97; 1960: Status of Local CORE groups, November 13, 1960, Series V: Departments and Related Organizations, No. 293, Reel 38, Frame 896; 1961: Affiliated CORE Groups list, October 10, 1961, Series II: Assistant to the National Director's File, No. 31, Reel 7, Frame 628; 1962: Organization Report, August 1, 1963, Series V: Departments and Related Organizations, No. 293, Reel 38, Frame 923; 1963: Affiliated CORE Chapters as of November 6, 1963, Series IV: National Action Council, No. 8, Reel 16, Frame 1295; 1964: Affiliated CORE Chapters, February 20, 1964, B: Associate National Director's Files, Series I, No. 32, Reel 9, Frame 92; 1965: Press Release: 16 new chapters affiliated, June 30, 1965, Series IV: National Action Council, No. 1, Reel 16, Frame 559.

Figure 5.7. 1960: 1960 Auditor's Report; 1961: Statement of Receipts and Expenditures for Fiscal Year Ending August 31, 1961; 1962: Auditor's Report for Fiscal Year Ending August 31, 1962; 1963: SCLC Annual Report; 1964: Income Statement, September 1, 1963–August 31, 1964; 1965: Financial Report Submitted to 9th Annual Convention, September 1, 1964–June 30, 1965; 1966: Audit Report for August 30, 1965–June 30,.

Figures 6.1, 6.2. NAACP Annual Reports, 1969–1975.

Figure 6.3. *Chapters source*: 1967: NUL, Part III: Records of the National Urban League, 1967–1979, Box 48, Number Full-Time Employees in Urban League, 1961–1967; 1968: NUL, Part III, Box 2, Whitney Young Address at 1970 Annual Conference, "Building Ghetto Power"; 1969: NUL, Part III, Box 14, Annual Report 1969; 1970: NUL, Part III, Box 1, Quarterly Affiliate Status, Summary, September 12, 1970; 1971: NUL, Part III, Box 2, July 28, 1971, Address by Vernon E. Jordan, ED-designate, NUL Conference; 1972: author's estimate; 1973: NUL, Part III, Box 14, Progress Report, 1973; 1974: NUL, Part III, Box 14, Annual Report, 1974. *Income source*: NUL Progress and Annual Reports, 1967–1974.

Bibliography

Aberbach, Joel D. and Bert A. Rockman. 2002. "Conducting and Coding Elite Interviews." *PS* (December): 673–76.

Abramovitz, Mimi. 2000. *Under Attack, Fighting Back: Women and Welfare in the United States.* New York: Monthly Review Press.

Ainsworth, Scott H. 2002. *Analyzing Interest Groups: Group Influence on People and Policies.* New York: Norton.

Axinn, June and Mark Stern. 2001. *Social Welfare: A History of the American Response to Need.* 5th ed. Boston: Allyn and Bacon.

Bacharach, Samuel B. and Edward J. Lawler. 1982. *Power and Politics in Organizations: The Social Psychology of Conflict, Coalitions, and Bargaining.* San Francisco: Jossey-Bass.

Bailis, Lawrence Neil. 1974. *Bread or Justice: Grassroots Organizing in the Welfare Rights Movement.* Toronto: Lexington Books.

Barakso, Maryann. 2004. *Governing NOW: Grassroots Activism in the National Organization for Women.* Ithaca, N.Y.: Cornell University Press.

———. 2005. "Civic Engagement and Voluntary Associations: Reconsidering the Role of the Governance Structures of Advocacy Groups." *Polity* 37, 3 (July): 315–34.

Barker, Lucius J., Mack H. Jones, and Katherine Tate. 1999. *African Americans and the American Political System.* Upper Saddle River, N.J.: Prentice-Hall.

Baumgartner, Frank R. and Beth L. Leech. 1998. *Basic Interests: The Importance of Groups in Politics and Political Science.* Princeton, N.J.: Princeton University Press.

Baumgartner, Frank R. and Beth L. Leech. 2001. "Interest Niches and Policy Bandwagons: Patterns of Interest Group Involvement in National Politics," *Journal of Politics* 63: 1191–1213.

Bayes, Jane H. 1982. *Minority Politics and Ideologies in the United States.* Novato, Calif.: Chandler and Sharp.

Bennett, Larry and Adolph Reed, Jr. 1999. "The New Face of Urban Renewal: The Near North Redevelopment Initiative and the Cabrini-Green Neighborhood." In *Without Justice for All: The New Liberalism and Our Retreat from Racial Equality,* ed. Adolph Reed, Jr. Boulder, Colo.: Westview Press.

Berkowitz, Edward D. 1991. *America's Welfare State: From Roosevelt to Reagan.* Baltimore: Johns Hopkins University Press.

Berry, Jeffrey M. 1984. *Interest Group Society*. Boston: Little Brown.

Berry, Jeffrey M., with David F. Arons. 2003. *A Voice for Non-Profits*. Washington, D.C.: Brookings Institution Press.

Berry, Jeffrey M., Kent E. Portney, and Ken Thomson. 1993. *The Rebirth of Urban Democracy*. Washington, D.C.: Brookings Institution.

Blank, Rebecca M. 1997. *It Takes a Nation: A New Agenda for Fighting Poverty*. Princeton, N.J.: Princeton University Press.

Bobo, Lawrence, and Franklin Gilliam. 1990. "Race, Sociopolitical Participation, and Black Empowerment." *American Political Science Review* 84, 2 (June): 377–93.

Bobo, Lawrence and Ryan A. Smith. 1998. "From Jim Crow Racism to Laissez-Faire Racism: The Transformation of Racial Attitudes." In *Beyond Pluralism: The Conception of Groups and Group Identities in America*, ed. Wendy F. Katkin, Ned Landsman, and Andrea Tyree. Urbana: University of Illinois Press.

Bok, Marcia. 1992. *Civil Rights and Social Programs of the 1960s: The Social Justice Functions of Social Policy*. Westport, Conn.: Praeger.

Bond, Julian. 2005. Foreword to Gilbert Jonas, *Freedom's Sword: The NAACP and the Struggle Against Racism in America, 1909–1969*. New York: Routledge.

Bond, Julian et al. 2009. *NAACP: Celebrating a Century*. Salt Lake City: Gibbs Smith.

Bracey, John H., Jr., and August Meier. 1995a. *Papers of the NAACP: Supplement to Part 1, 1956–1960*. Bethesda, Md.: University Publications of America.

———. 1995b. *Papers of the NAACP: Supplement to Part 1, 1961–1965*. Bethesda, Md.: University Publications of America.

———. 1995c. *Papers of the NAACP: Supplement to Part 4, Voting Rights, General Office Files, 1956–1965*. Bethesda, Md.: University Publications of America.

———. 1995d. *Papers of the NAACP: Supplement to Part 13, Labor Department Files, 1960–1965*. 1995e. *Papers of the NAACP: Supplement to Part 16, Board of Directors File, 1956–1965*. Bethesda, Md.: University Publications of America.

———. 1995f. *Papers of the NAACP: Supplement to Part 17, National Staff Files, 1956–1965*. Bethesda, Md.: University Publications of America.

———. 1995g. *Records of the Southern Christian Leadership Conference 1954–1970*. Bethesda, Md.: University Publications of America, 1995.

Browne, William P. 1990. "Organized Interests and Their Issue Niches: A Search for Pluralism in a Policy Domain." *Journal of Politics* 52, 2: 477–509.

———. 1998. *Groups, Interests, and U.S. Public Policy*. Washington, D.C.: Georgetown University Press.

Browning, Rufus P., Dale Rogers Marshall, and David H. Tabb. 1984. *Protest Is Not Enough: The Struggle of Blacks and Hispanics for Equality in Urban Politics*. Berkeley: University of California Press.

———. 1997. *Racial Politics in American Cities*. Berkeley: University of California Press.

Campbell, Andrea Louise. 2003. *How Policies Make Citizens: Senior Political Activism and the American Welfare State*. Princeton, N.J.: Princeton University Press.

Carmines, Edward and James Stimson. 1989. *Issue Evolution: Race and the Transformation of American Politics*. Princeton, N.J.: Princeton University Press.

Carson, Clayborne. 1995. *In Struggle: SNCC and the Black Awakening of the 1960s*. Cambridge, Mass.: Harvard University Press.

Cater, Douglass. 1964. *Power in Washington*. New York: Vintage Books.

Chase, Robert T. 1998. "Class Resurrection: The Poor People's Campaign of 1968 and Resurrection City," *Essays in History*, vol. 40, Virginia: The University of Virginia.

Childs, John Brown. 2007. *Hurricane Katrina: Response and Responsibilities*. 2nd ed. Berkeley, Calif.: North Atlantic Books.

Chong, Dennis. 1991. *Collective Action and the Civil Rights Movement*. Chicago: University of Chicago Press.

Clark, Kenneth. 1998. *A Relevant War Against Poverty: A Study of Community Action Programs and Observable Social Change*. New York: Metropolitan Applied Research Center.

Clark, Peter B. and James Q. Wilson. 1961. "Incentive Systems: A Theory of Organizations." *Administrative Science Quarterly* 6, 2: 129–61.

Clemens, Elisabeth S. 1997. *The People's Lobby: Organizational Innovation and the Rise of Interest Group Politics in the United States, 1890–1925*. Chicago: University of Chicago Press.

Cohen, Cathy J. 1999. *The Boundaries of Blackness*. Chicago: University of Chicago Press.

Cohen, Cathy J. and Michael C. Dawson. 1993. "Neighborhood Poverty and African American Politics." *American Political Science Review* 87, 2 (June): 286–302.

Collins, Sheila. 1996. *Let Them Eat Ketchup! The Politics of Poverty and Inequality*. New York: Monthly Review Press.

Congressional Quarterly. 1965. *Congress and the Nation*, Vol. 1, *1945–1964: A Review of Government and Politics in the Postwar Years*. Washington, D.C.: Congressional Research Service.

———. 1970. *Congress and the Nation*. Vol. 2, *1965–1968*. Washington, D.C.: Congressional Quarterly Service.

———. 1973. *Congress and the Nation*. Vol. 3, *1969–1972*. Washington, D.C.: Congressional Quarterly Service.

———. 1989. *Congress and the Nation*. Vol. 7, *1985–1988*. Washington, D.C.: Congressional Quarterly Service.

———. 1996. *Almanac: 104th Congress, 1st Session, 1995*, vol. 51. Washington, D.C.: Congressional Quarterly Service.

Conlan, Timothy. *From New Federalism to Devolution*. Washington, D.C.: Brookings Institution Press, 1998.

Dahl, Robert. 2005 [1961]. *Who Governs? Democracy and Power in an American City*. New Haven, Conn.: Yale University Press.

DaVita, Carol J. 1999. "Nonprofits and Devolution: What Do We Know?" In *Nonprofits and Government: Collaboration and Conflict*, ed. Elizabeth T. Boris and C. Eugene Steuerle. Washington, D.C.: Urban Institute Press.

Dawson, Michael. 1994. *Behind the Mule: Race and Class in African-American Politics*. Princeton, N.J.: Princeton University Press.

D'Emilio, John. 2003. *Lost Prophet: The Life and Times of Bayard Rustin*. New York: Free Press.

D'Emilio, John. 2004. "National Gay and Lesbian Task Force (NGLTF)." *Encyclopedia of Lesbian, Gay, Bisexual and Transgendered History in America*. Ed. Marc Stein. Vol. 2. Detroit: Gale. Northwestern University—CIC. Accessed by author on 16 June 2006.

Dickerson, Dennis C. 1998. *Militant Mediator: Whitney M. Young Jr.* Lexington, Ky.: University Press of Kentucky.

Dreier, Peter. 2006. "Katrina and Power in America," *Urban Affairs Review* 41: 528–49.

Dyson, Michael Eric. 2007. *Come Hell or High Water: Hurricane Katrina and the Color of Disaster*. New York: Civitas.

Eaklor, Vicky. 2004. "The Human Rights Campaign." *Encyclopedia of Lesbian,*

Gay, Bisexual and Transgendered History in America, ed. Marc Stein. Vol. 2. Detroit: Gale. Gale Virtual Reference Library. Thomson Gale. Northwestern University-CIC. Accessed 16 June 2006.

Edsall, Thomas B. and Mary D. Edsall. 1991. *Chain Reaction: The Impact of Race, Rights and Taxes on American Politics.* New York: Norton.

Fainstein, Norman I. and Susan S. Fainstein. 1974. *Urban Political Movements: The Search for Power by Minority Groups in American Cities.* Englewood Cliffs, N.J.: Prentice-Hall.

Fairclough, Adam. 1987. *To Redeem the Soul of America: The Southern Christian Leadership Conference and Martin Luther King Jr.* Athens: University of Georgia Press.

Feinberg, Leslie. 1996. *Transgender Warriors: Making History from Joan of Arc to RuPaul.* Boston: Beacon Press.

Flanagan, Richard M. 2001. "Lyndon Johnson, Community Action, and Management of the Administrative State." *Presidential Studies Quarterly* 31, 4 (December): 585–608.

Forman, James. 1997. *The Making of Black Revolutionaries.* Seattle: University of Washington Press.

Fraser, Nancy. 1993. "Clintonism, Welfare, and the Antisocial Wage: The Emergence of a Neoliberal Political Imaginary." *Rethinking Marxism* 6, 1: 10–19.

Frymer, Paul. 1999. *Uneasy Alliances: Race and Party Competition in America.* Princeton, N.J.: Princeton University Press.

———. 2008. *Black and Blue: African Americans, the Labor Movement, and the Decline of the Democratic Party.* Princeton, N.J.: Princeton University Press.

Frymer, Paul, Dara Z. Strolovitch, and Dorian Warren. 2006. "New Orleans Is Not the Exception: Re-Politicizing the Study of Racial Inequality." *DuBois Review* 3, 1: 37–57.

Gamson, William A. 1975. *The Strategy of Social Protest.* Homewood, Ill.: Dorsey Press.

Garrow, David J. 1986. *Bearing the Cross: Martin Luther King, Jr., and the Southern Christian Leadership Conference.* New York: W. Morrow.

Giddings, Paula. 1984. *When and Where I Enter: The Impact of Black Women on Race and Sex in America.* New York: Bantam.

Gilens, Martin. 1999. *Why Americans Hate Welfare: Race, Media and the Politics of Antipoverty Policy.* Chicago: University of Chicago Press.

Goldstein, Kenneth M. 1999. *Interest Groups, Lobbying, and Participation in America.* Cambridge: Cambridge University Press.

Goluboff, Risa L. 2007. *The Lost Promise of Civil Rights.* Cambridge, Mass.: Harvard University Press.

Gray, Virginia and David Lowery. 1996. *The Population Ecology of Interest Representation.* Ann Arbor: University of Michigan Press.

Greenstone, J. David. 1969. *Labor in American Politics.* New York: Alfred A. Knopf.

Hacker, Jacob S. 2002. *The Divided Welfare State: The Battle of Public and Private Social Benefits in the United States.* New York: Cambridge University Press.

Haines, Herbert H. 1988. *Black Radicals and the Civil Rights Mainstream, 1954–1970.* Knoxville: University of Tennessee Press.

Hamilton, Charles V. and Dona C. Hamilton. 1986. "Social Policies, Civil Rights, and Poverty." In *Fighting Poverty: What Works and What Doesn't,* ed. Sheldon H. Danziger and Daniel H. Weinberg. Cambridge, Mass.: Harvard University Press.

Hamilton, Dona C. and Charles V. Hamilton. 1992. "The Dual Agenda of African American Organizations Since the New Deal: Social Welfare Policies and Civil Rights." *Political Science Quarterly* 107, 3 (Autumn): 435–52.

————. 1997. *The Dual Agenda: Race and Social Welfare Policies of Civil Rights Organizations.* New York: Columbia University Press.

Hancock, Ange-Marie. 2004. *The Politics of Disgust: The Public Identity of the Welfare Queen.* New York: New York University Press.

Hardin, Russell. 1982. *Collective Action.* Baltimore: Johns Hopkins University Press.

Hays, R. Allen. 2001. *Who Speaks for the Poor: National Interest Groups and Social Policy.* New York: Routledge.

Heaney, Michael T. 2004. "Outside the Issue Niche: The Multidimensionality of Interest Group Identity." *American Politics Research* 32, 6: 611–51.

Heclo, Hugh. 1986. "The Political Foundations of Antipoverty Policy." In *Fighting Poverty: What Works and What Doesn't,* ed. Sheldon H. Danziger and Daniel H. Weinberg. Cambridge, Mass.: Harvard University Press.

Heclo, Hugh. 1978. "Issue Networks and the Executive Establishment." In *The New American Political System,* ed. Anthony King. Washington, D.C.: American Enterprise Institute.

Heinz, John P., Edward O. Laumann, Robert L. Nelson, and Robert H. Salisbury. 1993. *The Hollow Core: Private Interests in National Policy Making.* Cambridge, Mass.: Harvard University Press.

Hochschild, Jennifer. 1995. *Facing Up to the American Dream: Race, Class, and the Soul of the Nation.* Princeton, N.J.: Princeton University Press.

Hrebenar, Ronald J., and Ruth K. Scott. 1982. *Interest Group Politics in America.* Englewood Cliffs, N.J.: Prentice-Hall.

Jackson, Thomas F. 1993. "The State, the Movement, and the Urban Poor: The War on Poverty and Political Mobilization in the 1960s." In *The "Underclass" Debate: Views from History,* ed. Michael B. Katz. Princeton, N.J.: Princeton University Press.

————. 2007. *From Civil Rights to Human Rights: Martin Luther King, Jr., and the Struggle for Economic Justice.* Philadelphia: University of Pennsylvania Press.

Jacobs, Lawrence R., and Theda Skocpol. 2005. *Inequality and American Democracy: What We Know and What We Need to Learn.* New York: Sage.

Jennings, James. 1992. *The Politics of Black Empowerment: The Transformation of Black Activism in Urban America.* Detroit: Wayne State University Press.

Johnson, Ollie A. III and Karin L. Stanford, eds. 2002. *Black Political Organizations in the Post-Civil Rights Era.* New Brunswick, N.J.: Rutgers University Press.

Jonas, Gilbert. 2005. *Freedom's Sword: The NAACP and the Struggle Against Racism in America, 1909–1969.* New York: Routledge.

Jones, Jordy. 2004. "Transgender Organizations and Periodicals." *Encyclopedia of Lesbian, Gay, Bisexual and Transgendered History in America,* ed. Marc Stein. Vol. 3. Detroit: Gale, 2004. *Gale Virtual Reference Library.* Thomson Gale. Northwestern University-CIC. Accessed by author on 16 June 2006.

Kellogg, Charles Flint. 1967. *NAACP: A History of the National Association for the Advancement of Colored People.* Baltimore: Johns Hopkins University Press.

Kinder, Donald R. and Tali Mendelberg. 2000. "Individualism Reconsidered: Principles and Prejudice in Contemporary American Opinion." In *Racialized Politics: The Debate About Racism in America,* ed. David O. Sears, Jim Sidanius, and Lawrence Bobo. Chicago: University of Chicago Press.

Kinder, Donald R. and Lynn M. Sanders. 1996. *Divided by Color: Racial Politics and Democratic Ideals.* Chicago: University of Chicago Press.

Kollman, Ken. 1998. *Outside Lobbying: Public Opinion and Interest Group Strategies.* Princeton, N.J.: Princeton University Press.

Knoke, David. 1990. *Organizing for Collective Action: The Political Economies of Associations.* New York: Aldine de Gruyter.

Lieberman, Robert. *Shifting the Color Line: Race and the American Welfare State.* Cambridge, Mass.: Harvard University Press, 1998.

Lipset, Seymour Martin, Martin A. Trow, and James S. Coleman. 1956. *Union Democracy: The Internal Politics of the International Typographical Union.* Glencoe, Ill.: Free Press.

Lowi, Theodore J. 1969. *The End of Liberalism: The Second Republic of the United States.* New York: Norton.

Lynn, Laurence E., Jr. 1977. "A Decade of Policy Developments in the Income-Maintenance System." In *A Decade of Federal Antipoverty Programs: Achievements, Failures, and Lessons,* ed. Robert H. Haveman. New York: Academic Press.

Manley, John F. 1983. "Neo-Pluralism: A Class Analysis of Pluralism I and Pluralism II." *American Political Science Review* 77: 368–83.

Marable, Manning. 1985. *Black American Politics: From the Washington Marches to Jesse Jackson.* London: Verso.

Marable, Manning and Kristen Clarke, eds. 2008. *Seeking Higher Ground: The Hurricane Katrina Crisis, Race, and Public Policy Reader.* New York: Palgrave Macmillan.

March, James G., and Johan P. Olsen. 1989. *Rediscovering Institutions: The Organizational Basis of Politics.* New York: Free Press.

Marger, Martin N. 1984. "Social Movement Organizations and Response to Environmental Change: The NAACP, 1960–1973." *Social Problems* 32, 1 (October): 16–30.

Marris, Peter, and Martin Rein. 1973. *Dilemmas of Social Reform: Poverty and Community Action in the United States.* Chicago: Aldine.

Massey, Douglas S., and Nancy A. Denton. 1993. *American Apartheid: Segregation and the Making of the Underclass.* Cambridge, Mass.: Harvard University Press.

McAdam, Doug. 1982. *Political Process and the Development of Black Insurgency, 1930–1970.* Chicago: University of Chicago Press.

McConnell, Grant. 1966. *Private Power and American Democracy.* New York: Knopf.

McCarthy, John D. and Mayer N. Zald. 1973. *The Trend of Social Movements in America: Professionalization and Resource Mobilization.* Morristown, N.J.: General Learning Press.

McFarland, Andrew S. 1984. *Common Cause: Lobbying in the Public Interest.* Chatham, N.J.: Chatham House.

Meier, August and John H. Bracey, Jr. 1993. "The NAACP as Reform Movement, 1909–1965: 'To Reach the Conscience of America.'" *Journal of Southern History* 59 (February): 3–30.

Meier, August, and Elliott Rudwick. 1975 [1973]. *CORE: A Study in the Civil Rights Movement.* Oxford: Oxford University Press.

Michels, Robert. 1949. *Political Parties: A Sociological Study of the Oligarchical Tendencies of Modern Democracy.* Trans. Eden Paul and Cedar Paul. Glencoe, Ill.: Free Press.

Mink, Gwendolyn. 1998. *Welfare's End.* Ithaca, N.Y.: Cornell University Press, 1998.

———, ed. 1999. *Whose Welfare.* Ithaca, N.Y.: Cornell University Press, 1999.

Moe, Terry M. 1980. *The Organization of Interests: Incentives and the Internal Dynamics of Political Interest Groups.* Chicago: University of Chicago Press.

Moore, Jesse Thomas. 1981. *A Search for Equality: The National Urban League, 1910–1961.* University Park: Pennsylvania State University Press.

Morris, Aldon. 1984. *The Origins of the Civil Rights Movement: Black Communities Organizing for Change.* New York: Free Press.

NAACP. 1966. *NAACP Annual Report 1965.* New York: NAACP.

Nadasen, Premilla. 2005. *Welfare Warriors: The Welfare Rights Movement in the United States.* New York, N.Y.: Routledge.

Naples, Nancy A. 1998. *Grassroots Warriors: Activist Mothering, Community Work, and the War on Poverty.* New York: Routledge.

Noble, Charles. 1997. *Welfare as We Knew It: A Political History of the American Welfare State.* New York: Oxford University Press.

Olson, Mancur. 1965. *The Logic of Collective Action: Public Goods and the Theory of Groups.* Cambridge, Mass.: Harvard University Press.

Oliver, Melvin L. and Thomas M. Shapiro. 1995. *Black Wealth/White Wealth: A New Perspective on Racial Inequality.* New York: Routledge.

Omi, Michael and Howard Winant. 1994. *Racial Formation in the United States: From the 1960s to the 1990s.* New York: Routledge.

Parris, Guichard and Lester Brooks. 1971. *Blacks in the City: A History of the National Urban League.* Toronto: Little, Brown.

Patterson, James T. 1994. *America's Struggle Against Poverty 1900–1994.* Cambridge, Mass.: Harvard University Press.

Pattillo-McCoy, Mary. 1999. *Black Picket Fences: Privilege and Peril Among the Black Middle Class.* Chicago: University of Chicago Press, 1999.

Peake, Thomas R. 1987. *Keeping the Dream Alive: A History of the Southern Christian Leadership Conference from King to the Nineteen-Eighties.* New York: Peter Lang.

Peterson, Paul E. 1981. *City Limits.* Chicago: University of Chicago Press.

Piven, Frances Fox and Richard A. Cloward. 1977. *Poor People's Movements: Why They Succeed and How They Fail.* New York: Pantheon.

———. 1993 [1971]. *Regulating the Poor: The Functions of Public Welfare.* New York: Vintage.

Polletta, Francesca. 2004. *Freedom Is an Endless Meeting: Democracy in American Social Movements.* Chicago: University of Chicago Press.

Quadagno, Jill. 1992. "Social Movements and State Transformation: Labor Unions and Racial Conflict in the War on Poverty." *American Sociological Review* 57, 5 (October): 616–34.

———. 1994. *The Color of Welfare: How Racism Undermined the War on Poverty.* New York: Oxford University Press.

Ransby, Barbara. 2003. *Ella Baker and the Black Freedom Movement.* Chapel Hill: University of North Carolina Press.

Reed, Adolph. 1999. *Stirrings in the Jug: Black Politics in the Post-Segregation Era.* Minneapolis: University of Minnesota Press.

Reed, Christopher Robert. 1997. *The Chicago NAACP and the Rise of Black Professional Leadership 1910–1966.* Bloomington: Indiana University Press.

Reid, Elizabeth J. 1999. "Nonprofit Advocacy and Political Participation." In *Nonprofits and Government: Collaboration and Conflict,* ed. Elizabeth T. Boris and C. Eugene Steuerle. Washington, D.C.: Urban Institute Press.

Rhym, Darren. 2002. *The NAACP.* Philadelphia: Chelsea House.

Rich, Marvin. 1965. "The Congress of Racial Equality of Its Strategy." *Annals of the American Academy of Political and Social Science* 357, 1: 113–18.

Robnett, Belinda. 2000. *How Long? How Long?: African American Women in the Struggle for Civil Rights.* Oxford: Oxford University Press.

Rosenstone, Steven J. and John Mark Hansen. 1993. *Mobilization, Participation, and Democracy in America.* New York: Macmillan.

Ross, Robert L. 1970. "Relations Among National Interest Groups." *Journal of Politics* 32, 1 (February): 96–114.

Rothenberg, Lawrence S. 1992. *Linking Citizens to Government: Interest Group Politics at Common Cause.* New York: Cambridge University Press.

Rudwick, Elliott, and August Meier. 1970. "Organizational Structure and Goal Succession: A Comparative Analysis of the NAACP and CORE, 1964–1968." *Social Science Quarterly* 51 (June): 9–24.

Salisbury, Robert H. 1969. "An Exchange Theory of Interest Groups." *Midwest Journal of Political Science* 13, 1 (February): 1–32.

Salisbury, Robert H. 1984. "Interest Representation: The Dominance of Institutions." *American Political Science Review,* 78, 1 (March): 64–76.

Schattschneider, E. E. 1960. *The Semisovereign People: A Realist's View of Democracy in America.* New York: Holt, Rinehart.

Schlozman, Kay Lehman and John T. Tierney. 1986. *Organized Interests and American Democracy.* New York: Harper and Row.

Schuman, Howard et al. 1997. *Racial Attitudes in America: Trends and Interpretations.* Cambridge, Mass.: Harvard University Press.

Sellers, Cleveland with Robert Terrell. 1990. *The River of No Return: the Autobiography of a Black Militant and the Life and Death of SNCC.* Jackson: University of Mississippi Press.

Sigleman, Lee and Susan Welch. 1994. *Black Americans' Views of Racial Inequality: The Dream Deferred.* Cambridge: Cambridge University Press.

Singh, Robert. 1998. *The Congressional Black Caucus: Racial Politics in the U.S. Congress.* Thousand Oaks, Calif.: Sage.

Skocpol, Theda. 2003. *Diminished Democracy: From Membership to Management in American Civic Life.* Norman: University of Oklahoma Press.

Smith, Robert C. 2002. "The NAACP in the Twenty-First Century." In *Black Political Organizations in the Post-Civil Rights Era,* ed. Ollie A. Johnson, III, and Karin L. Stanford. New Brunswick, N.J.: Rutgers University Press.

Smith, Sally Bedell. 2007. *For the Love of Politics: Inside the Clinton White House.* New York: Random House.

Steinberg, Stephen. 1995. *Turning Back: The Retreat from Racial Justice in American Thought and Policy.* Boston: Beacon Press.

Stone, Clarence, and Carol Perannuzi. 1997. "Atlanta and the Limited Reach of Electoral Control." In *Racial Politics in American Cities,* ed. Rufus P. Browning, Dale Rogers Marshall, and David H. Tabb. New York: Longman.

Stoper, Emily. 1989. *The Student Nonviolent Coordinating Committee: The Growth of Radicalism in a Civil Rights Organization.* Brooklyn, N.Y.: Carlson.

Strolovitch, Dara Z. 2006. "Do Interest Groups Represent the Disadvantaged? Advocacy at the Intersections of Race, Class, and Gender." *Journal of Politics* 68, 4: 894–910.

———. 2007. *Affirmative Advocacy: Race, Class, and Gender in Interest Group Politics.* Chicago: University of Chicago Press.

Tarrow, Sidney. 1994. *Power in Movement: Social Movements, Collective Action and Politics.* Cambridge: Cambridge University Press.

Teles, Steven M. 1996. *Whose Welfare? AFDC and Elite Politics.* Lawrence: University Press of Kansas.

Tierney, John. 1994. "Interest Group Research: Questions and Approaches." In *Representing Interests and Interest Group Representation,* ed. William Crotty, Mildred A. Schwartz, and John C. Green. Akron, Ohio: Ray C. Bliss Institute of Applied Politics.

Tate, Katherine. 1994. *From Protest to Politics: The New Black Voters in American Elections.* Cambridge, Mass.: Harvard University Press.

Truman, David B. 1960 [1951]. *The Governmental Process.* New York: Knopf.

Verba, Sidney, Kay Lehman Schlozman, and Henry E. Brady. 1995. *Voice and Equality: Civic Voluntarism in American Politics.* Cambridge, Mass.: Harvard University Press.

————. 1997. "The Big Tilt: Participatory Inequality in America." *American Prospect* 32: 74–80.

Walker, Jack L., Jr. 1991. *Mobilizing Interest Groups in America: Patrons, Professions, and Social Movements.* Ann Arbor: University of Michigan Press.

Weaver, R. Kent. 2000. *Ending Welfare as We Know It.* Washington, D.C.: Brookings Institution.

Weir, Margaret. 1993. "From Equal Opportunity to 'The New Social Contract': Race and the Politics of the American 'Underclass'." In *Racism, the City, and the State,* ed. Malcolm Cross and Michael Keith. New York: Routledge, 1993.

West, Guida. 1981. *The National Welfare Rights Movement: The Social Protest of Poor Women.* New York: Praeger.

Wilkins, Roy. 1994 [1982]. *Standing Fast: The Autobiography of Roy Wilkins,* New York: Da Capo Press.

Wilson, James Q. 1995 [1973]. *Political Organizations.* Princeton, N.J.: Princeton University Press.

Wilson, William Julius. *The Truly Disadvantaged: The Inner City, the Underclass, and Public Policy.* Chicago: University of Chicago Press.

————. 1996. *When Work Disappears: The World of the New Urban Poor.* New York: Knopf.

Zald, Mayer N., and Roberta Ash Garner. 1987. "Social Movement Organizations: Growth, Decay, and Change." In *Social Movements in an Organizational Society,* ed. Mayer N. Zald and John D. McCarthy. New Brunswick, N.J.: Transaction Books.

Zald, Mayer N., and John D. McCarthy. 1987. "Social Movement Industries: Competition and Conflict among SMOs." In *Social Movements in an Organizational Society,* ed. Mayer N. Zald and John D. McCarthy. New Brunswick, N.J.: Transaction Books.

Zinn, Howard. 1965. *SNCC: The New Abolitionists.* Boston: Beacon Press, 1965.

Hamilton, Charles, 8
Hamilton, Dona, 8
Haynes, George E., 16
Hill, Herbert, 45
Hill, Norman, 55–56
Hurricane Katrina, 1, 5, 6, 145–57; NAACP
 response, 146–53; NUL response,
 153–57; organizational response, 2
Hutchinson, Earl Ofari, 1

Innis, Roy, 122
Interest groups: competition, 33–35; decision making, 7; elite influence, 35–36;
 establishment, 10; external influences,
 12, 33–36; factors influencing priorities,
 9–10, 28–37; ideology, 10; internal
 influences, 12, 31–32; issue niches, 34;
 membership, 29–31; purposive groups,
 29

Jones, Eugene K., 16
Jordan, Vernon, 87, 129; testimony against
 Family Assistance Plan, 87

King, Martin Luther, Jr., 60, 62
Ku Klux Klan, 15

Lafayette, Bernard, 64
Lewis, John, 2, 68
Linked racial fate, 3

McCain, James, 17
McClain, Richard W., 77
McKissick, Floyd, 58, 110
Mitchell, Clarence, testimony on Family
 Assistance Plan, 80, 81
Morial, Marc, 154, 156
Morris, Jesse, 70
Moynihan Report, 40; civil rights response,
 40

NAACP. *See* National Association for the
 Advancement of Colored People
National Association for the Advancement
 of Colored People (NAACP): affiliate
 response to Hurricane Katrina, 149–50,
 152–53; archives, 171–73, 185n6; attention to anti-poverty policy, 90 (tab.);
 attention to Hurricane Katrina, 136
 (fig.); attention to TANF reform, 136
 (fig.); Black Nationalism, 121; branches,

125, 125 (fig.); foundation funding,
 186n13, 203n19; founding, 13–15, 21,
 21 (tab.); income, 98–99, 99 (fig.), 124,
 124 (fig.); membership, 8, 15, 98–99, 99
 (fig.), 125, 125 (fig.); position on Economic Opportunity Act, 41 (tab.); relations with branches, 14–15, 97–99;
 relations with Nixon administration, 81;
 relations with unions, 186n11; response
 to 1967 Amendments to Economic
 Opportunity Act, 77–79; response to
 Family Assistance Plan, 79–82; response
 to Hurricane Katrina, 146–53; response
 to Social Security Act Amendments, 44;
 response to state welfare laws, 42;
 response to TANF reform, 137–40;
 response to War on Poverty, 9, 44–46;
 role among civil rights organizations,
 97–99, 119–23; structure, 1, 12, 96–97,
 124–26, 137, 140, 150; testimony on
 Family Assistance Plan, 189n17
National League for Protection of Colored
 Women, 15
National League on Urban Conditions
 Among Negroes, 15
National Negro Conference, 13
National Urban League (NUL): 1963 reorganization, 102; archives, 173, 185n6;
 attention to anti-poverty policy, 90
 (tab.); attention to Hurricane Katrina,
 136 (fig.); attention to TANF reform,
 136 (fig.); budget, 101; Central Planning Unit, 131; chapters, 101 (fig.), 130,
 130 (fig.); Community Action Assembly,
 51; Domestic Marshall Plan, 46, 86;
 foundation funding, 204n26; founding,
 15–16, 21, 21 (tab.); guaranteed income
 plan, 85; income, 101 (fig.), 130, 130
 (fig.); Katrina Bill of Rights, 153–55;
 membership, 101; New Thrust Initiative,
 84, 126–29, 130–33; position on Economic Opportunity Act, 41 (tab.); relations to local offices, 16, 50–51, 101–2;
 relations with Johnson administration,
 49–50, 51, 52; relations with Nixon
 administration, 85; relations with OEO,
 50–52, 99; response to 1967 Amendments to Economic Opportunity Act,
 82–84; response to Family Assistance
 Plan, 85–88; response to Hurricane
 Katrina, 153–57; response to Newburgh

Acknowledgments

I am very grateful to have had the support of family, friends, and colleagues throughout the many years this project has endured. I am exceedingly thankful for their insights, patience, and support throughout this process. Most important, I would like to thank the civil rights leaders and staff who were interviewed for this project. I was very fortunate to speak with people who have committed their lives to effecting change within the American democratic system. Each leader and staff person, despite very demanding schedules that often remain devoted to securing civil rights in the United States, was kind enough to take time to speak with me and even follow-up over e-mail. I am very grateful for their generosity with their time and ideas.

Dennis Chong, Reuel R. Rogers, and Benjamin I. Page have been highly engaged in this project. I have been fortunate to learn a great deal from each of them. Ben has influenced my understanding of American politics and my research choices, challenging my assumptions and asking provoking questions. I thank him for his support of the project.

Reuel Rogers's scholarly perspective on race and representation shaped this research from its beginning stages. He encouraged me to interrogate how a sense of linked racial fate might translate into political representation; his encouragement was always accompanied by thoughtful, and thought-provoking, questions and comments. Reuel has read and commented on chapters, offering valuable advice and feedback. I thank him for his help and advice throughout the years, and for his constant reminders not to forget the questions that generated my interest in my research topic.

Dennis Chong's contributions to this project are immeasurable. I appreciate his openness to my project, and the rigorous standards to which he holds my research. Dennis's advice took the form of comments on written work, critiques of presentation, late night phone-consultations about my research, and even advice about financial planning for research costs. His comments and advice were always challenging to address, but also made the research and writing process very rewarding. I thank Dennis for his contributions to this research.

I am very grateful to have the support of my colleagues at Simmons College. Beginning in my first year, they have consistently encouraged my research agenda. Zachary Abuza is a model of a teacher-scholar. Since I arrived at Simmons, Zach has been helpful, particularly with advice on managing a research and teaching balance. I appreciate Kirk Beattie's friendly inquiries about my research and encouragement as I moved forward with this project. Carole Biewener's commitment to issues of social justice is inspiring, and I have benefitted from her keen insights about my project and the applicability of its findings. A special thank you to Cheryl Welch, who offered to read a chapter at a particularly important point in my writing process. Her feedback and advice were insightful and helped me move forward with the project. Diane Raymond has offered consistent encouragement of my research. I thank her for modeling, and supporting, a commitment to research within a small liberal arts college. Leanne Doherty has patiently listened as I wrestle with research frustrations, and then asked one or two questions that allowed me to figure out answers myself. I especially thank Leanne for her friendship and support.

My research took me to many libraries, and I was fortunate to be generously helped by knowledgeable staff at each one. I thank the staff of the Periodicals rooms at the Northwestern library, the University of Chicago Library, and Roosevelt University Library. Also, thank you to the staff of the Vivian G. Harsh Research Collection of Afro-American History and Literature at the Carter G. Woodson Regional Library in Chicago. I appreciate the help and competence of the staff of the Library of Congress Manuscript Reading Room. The Library of Congress staff were not only friendly about sharing their extensive knowledge of the archives, but was equally helpful when I continually asked for photocopying permission.

I was fortunate to receive fellowship and grant support to research and write this project. The Graduate School at Northwestern University provided research funding through a Graduate Research Grant. I also received research support from the MacArthur Fund in the Political Science Department and a Research Grant from the Legal Studies Program, both at Northwestern. The Alan and Sherry Leventhal Fellowship in the Graduate School at Northwestern University provided support for research and writing. After I arrived at Simmons College, funding from the Simmons Fund for Faculty Research allowed me to complete interviews with organizational leaders and staff.

Careful readings and comments by colleagues throughout the years have helped me sharpen questions and re-think findings. I am very grateful for the insights of: Maryann Barakso, Rebecca Givan, Michael Hanchard, Melissa Harris-Lacewell, Kerry Haynie, Ken Janda, Jane Junn, Natalie Masuoka, Andrea Simpson, Lester Kenyatta Spence, Dara Strolovitch, and Dorian Warren. I thank Peter Agree at the University of Pennsylvania Press for his consistent support and enthusiasm for this book. Rick Valelly, one of the editors of this series, has provided insightful feedback and excitement about this book since our first conversations about my research. I thank him for including my book in a series that seeks to analyze American democracy from a problem-based approach. This book benefitted greatly from the comments, criticisms, and insights provided by two anonymous reviewers. I thank both reviewers for their careful readings of my book. I also thank the editors at the *DuBois Review* for permission to publish pieces of this project, which appeared in the Fall 2008 volume.

This project has benefited from input from friends, both within, and outside of, academic circles. Brandon Rottinghaus helped me shape my initial research questions, read conference papers and drafts, asked insightful questions—his input continues to anchor my ideas in scholarly questions raised in American politics research. Dan Bergan, Rebecca Givan, Dukhong Kim, Natalie Masuoka, and Adam Silver also gave me valuable comments about the project. I thank them for their input and friendship. I have found the insights of friends outside of academia to be particularly helpful, especially as I grappled with the "so what?" questions in my research. Over breakfasts, coffees, and dinners, they listened to me talk about my work, asked questions, and helped me think about the "bigger picture." Laura Gitelson has been engaged with this project since its inception. I thank her for her patience, questions, and advice. Heather Johnson has offered consistent intellectual and emotional support throughout the research and writing processes. I thank Heather for her intellectual engagement with my project, which included many late nights editing drafts of chapters.

While they may not have read chapters, my friends and family have been patient and supportive, even as I avoided phone calls and e-mails to finish coding data or writing a chapter. I thank my brother, Will Paden, for his interest in this project and his overall support. I am grateful to my friends and family for their encouragement throughout this process: Frances Freeman, Jean Freeman, John Newlin, Lee and Cliff Freeman, Zach Abuza, Barbara Becker, Leanne Doherty, Jason Evans, Ruth Fasoldt, Idy and Alan Gitelson, Rachel Gitelson, Becky Givan, Adrienne Hines, Ray and Jennifer Johnson, Patrice Johnson, Stephanie Jones, Suzanne Leonard, Tracy LeRoy, Adrienne and Syd Lieberman, Natalie Masuoka, Adam Silver, and Sarah Lieberman Weisz.

Finally, this book is dedicated to my parents, Fran and Bill Paden. My parents have offered incredible support for this book—they have talked me through research questions, read chapters at the very last minute, and offered insight when I became intellectually frustrated. My appreciation for their support extends far beyond this book, however. I was raised in an academic household where a commitment to pursuing intellectual curiosities was ingrained from an early age. More exceptionally, my brother and I were raised with an understanding of the importance of questioning norms and acting when we did not like the answers. I thank them for values they instilled through belief and action. Finally, I thank them for their confidence in me.

The insight I have received from mentors, colleagues, and friends has shaped my approach to the topic of civil rights and poverty advocacy and in the United States. Of course, any errors are my own.